BODY AND SOUL

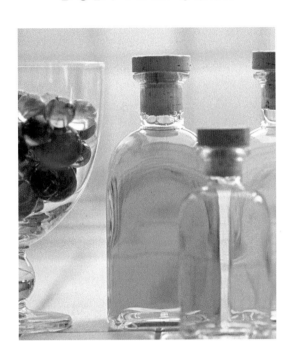

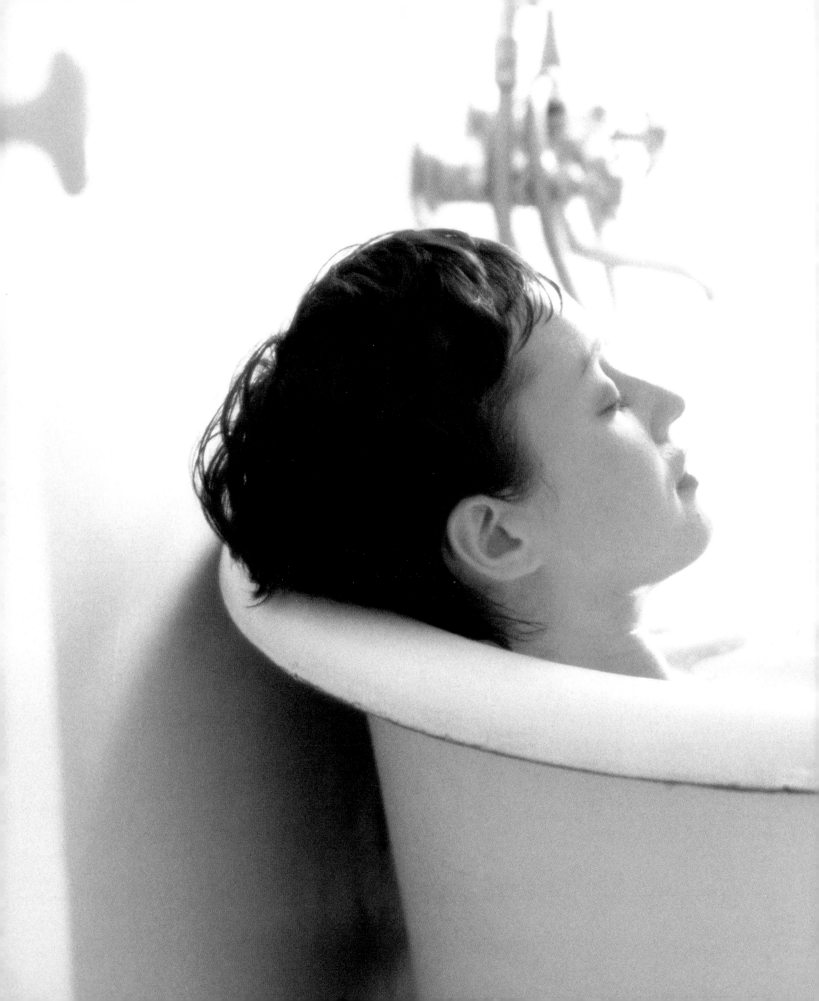

MIREILLE JOCHUM-GUILLOU   WERNER WALDMANN

BODY AND SOUL

CREATE YOUR OWN SPA

IN COOPERATION WITH
GERTRUD TEUSEN AND EDGAR GUGENHAN

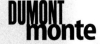

Conception and realisation: MediText, Stuttgart
Text: Mireille Jochum-Guillou, Werner Waldmann
Translation: Beate Gorman
Copy editing: Andrew Leslie
Layout: Karolina Stuhec Meglic
Photographs: cover: Photo Alto; other photographs: Adobe Image Library (8); Bäder
Obermaier (8); CMA (10); Creativ Collection (2); Deutscher Sauna Bund (1); Digital
Stock (1); Digital Vision (4); Duravit (14); Emco Erwin Müller Gruppe Lingen (1);
Good Shoot (3); hansgrohe (5); Hansgrohe Historisches Archiv (2); Ideal-Standard (4);
IKEA (4); Image 100 (2); Image Source (1); Kaldewei (1); Klafs Saunabau (2); MEV (2);
Museum Rietberg, Zürich (2); Photo Alto (24); Photo Disc (20); Sammlung Waldmann
(4); Schwarzkopf & Henkel Cosmetics (1); Sertürner (2); Stockbyte (2); Universitäts-
bibliothek Heidelberg (1); Universitätsbibliothek Leipzig (1); Villeroy & Boch (13);
Werner Waldmann (69)
Data management: DDS Lenhard, Stuttgart

Printing: Appl, Wemding (Germany)

© 2001 DuMont Buchverlag, Köln
(Dumont monte, UK, London)

ISBN 3-7701-7027-X
Printed in Germany

For more detailed information on the topics of bathing and well-being, please
contact the authoress Mireille Jochum-Guillou:
Thalasso Plus ®
International headquarters
Tel.: +49/6 81/3 90 69 65
Fax: +49/6 81/37 24 56
Kaiserstr. 7
66111 Saarbrücken

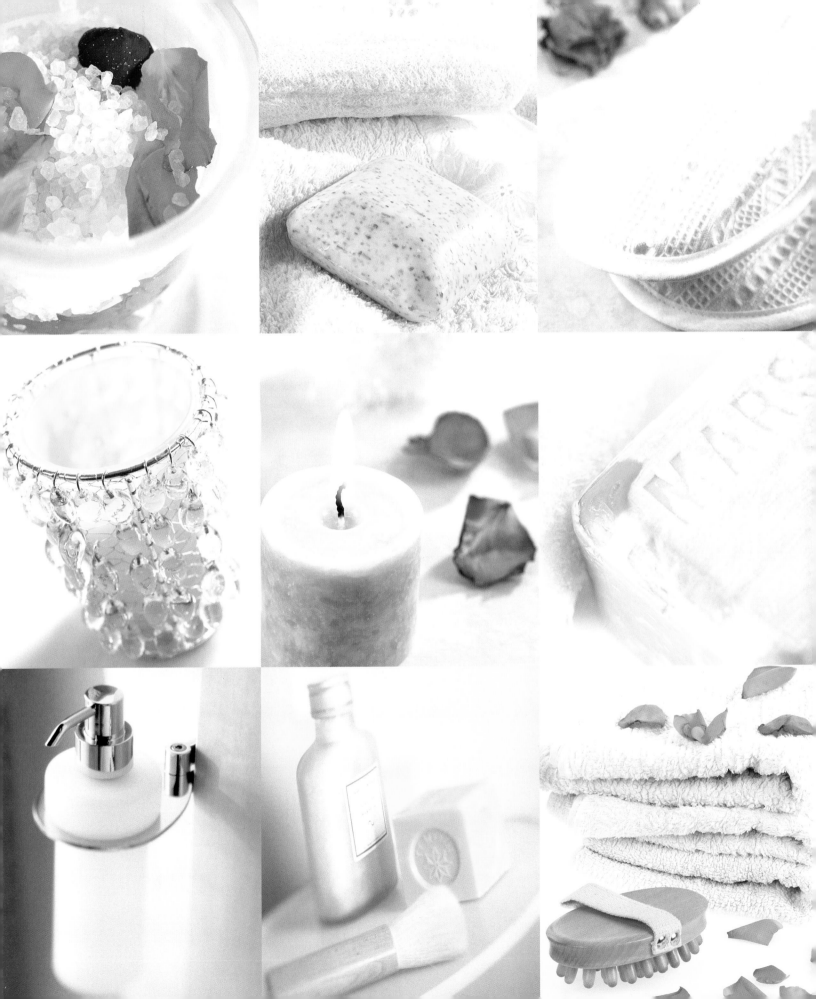

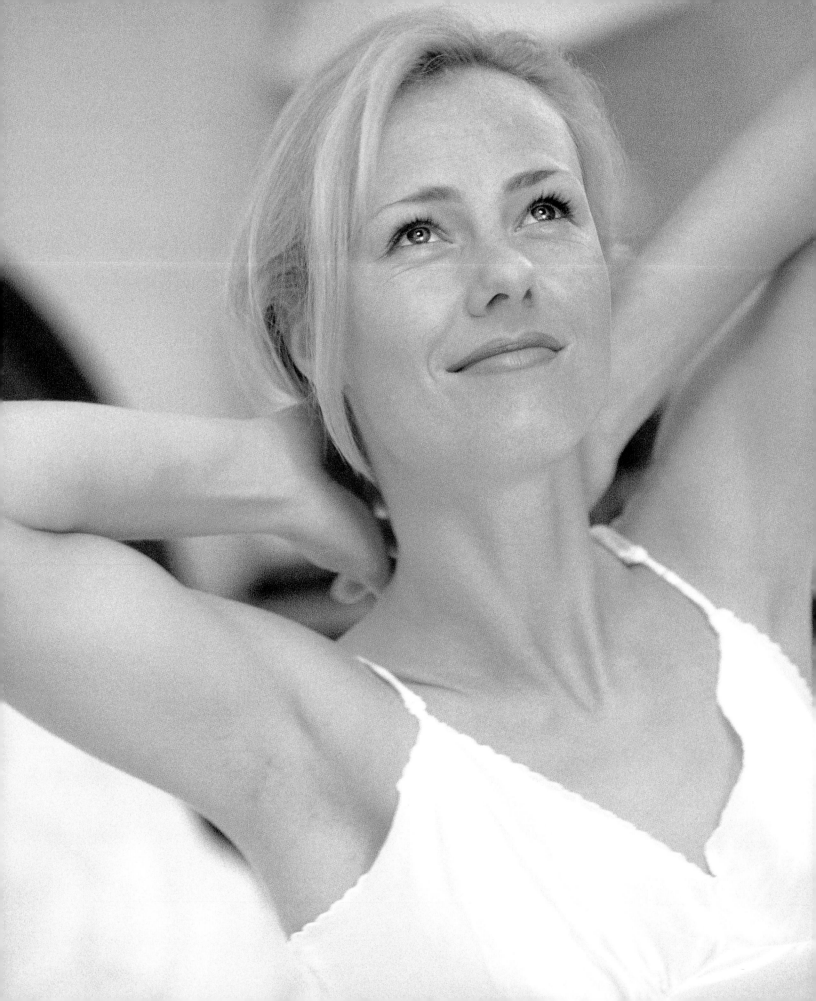

ON FEELING GOOD

Feeling good means being absolutely content with yourself, feeling happy and at peace with the world. Feeling good takes in the body and the soul to an equal extent. Your body is well organised, causes you no annoyance, you have no pain and absolutely no thoughts of taking medication. You are pleased with your appearance, enjoy looking in the mirror and perhaps even admire yourself. Feeling good is also related to striking an inner balance. People who *feel good* have no problems – and if they do acquire some, they are able to distance themselves from them easily.

For some, feeling good may have something to do with success in one's job or private life, while for others, health is an indispensable ingredient of well-being. There are still other people who only feel good when they are satisfied with their appearance and with their body in general.

Of course, everyone understands well-being in a slightly different way. Let us agree that we feel good when we are able to shrug off the day-to-day humdrum routine and the demands it brings with it as soon as we enter our own home, like hanging up a heavy burden in the wardrobe, and simply enjoy ourselves with no time constraints.

THE PATH TO WELL-BEING

In order to do something for our body, we also have to make our psyche work. If you have had a long, strenuous day at the office and were faced with a number of unpleasant situations, simply step under the hot shower as soon as you get home, hold your hands and face under the running water for several minutes and cleanse your body with a pleasantly fragrant shower gel. After this, enjoy a massage and mix yourself a refreshing drink – you will soon find that you feel much better than you did a few hours ago. Your organism suddenly switches over, and relaxation spreads throughout your body. Gentle, soothing music, the smell of fresh flowers, your skin feeling warm and this smell of freshness all around you – you feel clean, and your body is free of waste products. You could also say you have reached a state of well-being.

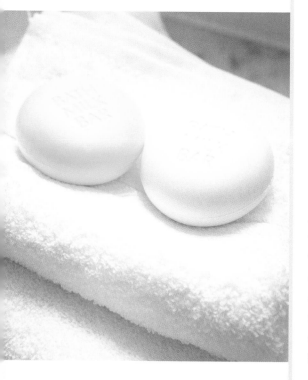

Feeling good is not something you can simply buy – you have to make a conscious effort. And it is not expensive. However, you will require a certain strategy to achieve this lovely, relaxing sensation.

The Bathroom – a Place to Spoil Yourself

Not too long ago, no one considered the subject of bathrooms worthy of serious discussion. The bathroom was more or less the "wet cell" used to maintain a minimum level of hygiene. And this unsightly small room was also used for brushing your teeth, washing your face and hands, shaving and putting on makeup. You could wash yourself more comfortably in the shower recess shielded by a plastic curtain than standing at the sink with a flannel and soap. Those who had sufficient space also had a bath, where they could sit and splash around. And apart from this, the bathroom was often used as a storage room where all sorts of rubbish could be kept out of sight and out of mind. This did not even disturb the people with their usual washing ritual. Apparently, some people's bathrooms were even cluttered with objects that had to be cleared out every week before the Saturday evening bath.

Occasionally, other types of bathrooms could be seen at the cinema or in weekly magazines. These had the dimensions of enormous living rooms and would have been more at home in a palace. The average person was not in the least envious; after all, they thought it very strange indeed that the humble bathroom should be furnished more luxuriously than the rest of the house.

But in the meantime, a complete transformation has taken place. People discovered the bathroom because they found out that bathing can be an important factor in their sense of well-being – this is something that cannot be explained away by hygiene alone.

Practically every culture has its own bathing tradition. The Romans were absolutely obsessed with bathing as a social event. But in the Middle Ages, too, people had their fun with water. At home, people from every social class treated themselves to the delights of bathing in a wooden tub of water. In public, they met in the bathhouses – men and women together – where they had a lot of fun. If we believe the stories that have been passed down, much fun indeed. However, epidemics and the Church soon put an end to this.

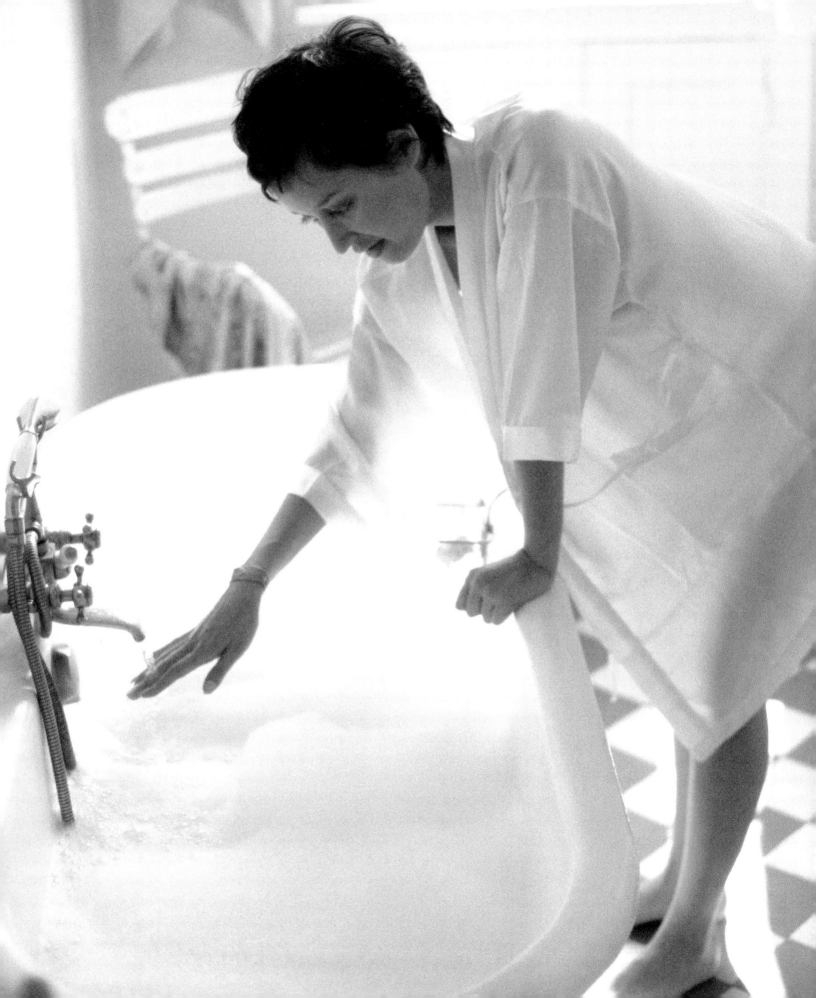

For the Japanese, bathing is almost a religious act that is by no means only a matter of hygiene – on the contrary. Before a Japanese steps into a private or shared bath, he washes himself thoroughly. In Japan, it would be unthinkable to have a bath when the body is not clean. The purpose of a bath is to cleanse the *soul*.

Over the years, bathrooms have become quite a respectable place throughout the Western world. Now, apart from the body, the soul can also be cleansed. Bathroom designers offer remarkable collections of baths, shower cabinets, basins, mirrored cabinets and fittings. People have at last realised that shape, colour and light play a significant role in creating an atmosphere in the bathroom that allows one to slip into the realm of dreams in the foamy bathwater.

The cosmetic industry has borrowed many ideas from nature. Although bath additives, essential oils, soaps, lotions, masks and exfoliants are manufactured on an industrial scale, nature invented the ingredients a long time ago. We can utilise the healing powers of spices, herbs and the sea at home to provide beauty, health and vitality. It is fascinating to consider just what an arsenal of materials we have at our fingertips to reunite body, mind and spirit.

Luxury as a Reward and Therapy

Those who still cling to the puritanical view that the bathroom should be used exclusively for washing and brushing their teeth may pass harsh

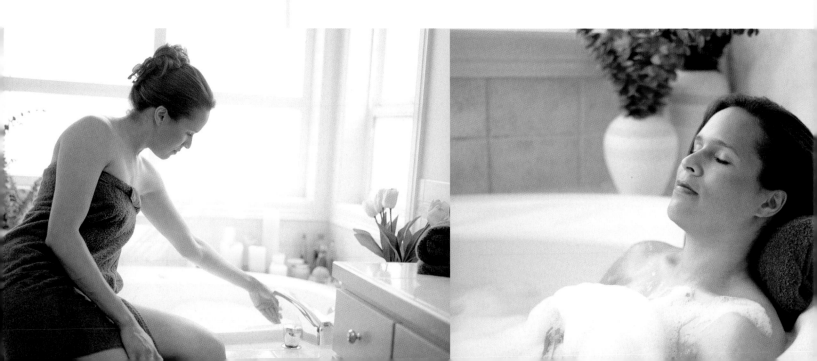

judgement on all the gadgetry to be found these days in bathrooms. New houses are being equipped not just with wonderfully designed bathrooms but also with spas and intricate baths which, in the past, would have been ascribed to the fantasy of a Hollywood prop designer. The shelves are filled with an assortment of bottles and flasks containing oils and essences. That is luxury, pure luxury. But isn't luxury the privilege of the upper ten thousand? No, it isn't – luxury is like salt in your soup. You don't need too much of it, but you can't do without it. If you work and are subjected to stress you also need relaxation and pleasure. Anything that can provide us with a zest for living is legitimate, including the ritual of spoiling ourselves in the bathroom, the cosmetic treatment or an exquisite culinary adventure. Beauty, being well groomed, and pleasure – these three elements bring the body into harmony with the mind and spirit, enrich the emotions and generate new energy for work and commitment.

When we spoil ourselves, we stimulate an enormous amount of power within us that provides us with quality of life, helps the body resist illness and strengthens creativity and vitality.

This book will show you many ways of pampering your body and soul. So simply relax and abandon yourself to pleasure.

Mireille Jochum-Guillou
Werner Waldmann

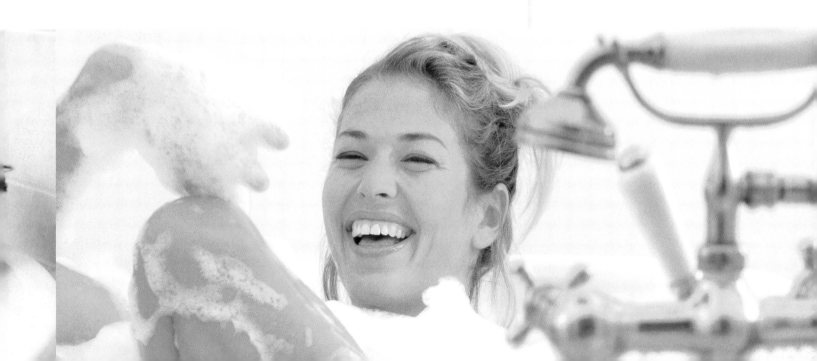

CONTENTS

A BRIEF HISTORY OF BATHING CULTURE 15

BATH ESSENTIALS 35

99 BATH ADDITIVES FOR YOUR WELL-BEING 63

A PROGRAMME FOR SPOILING YOURSELF 101

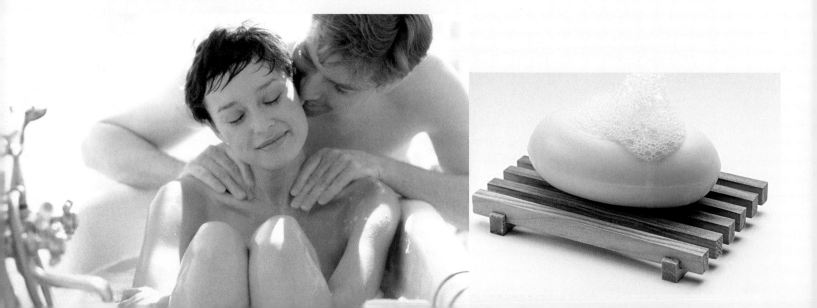

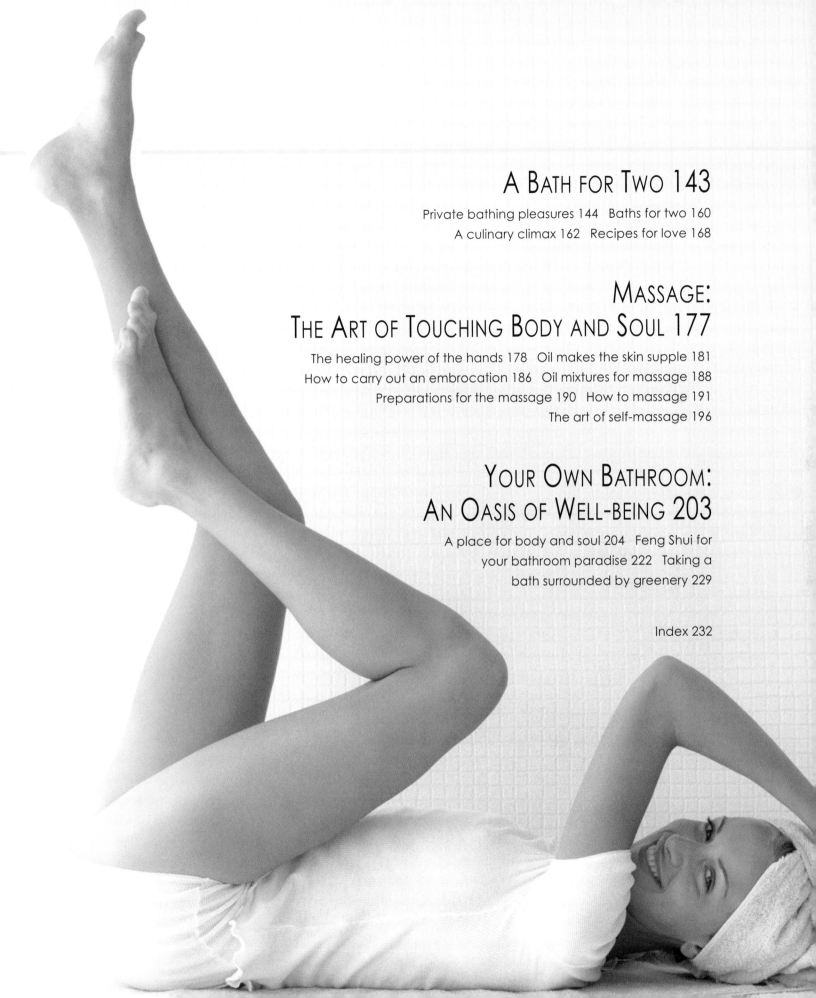

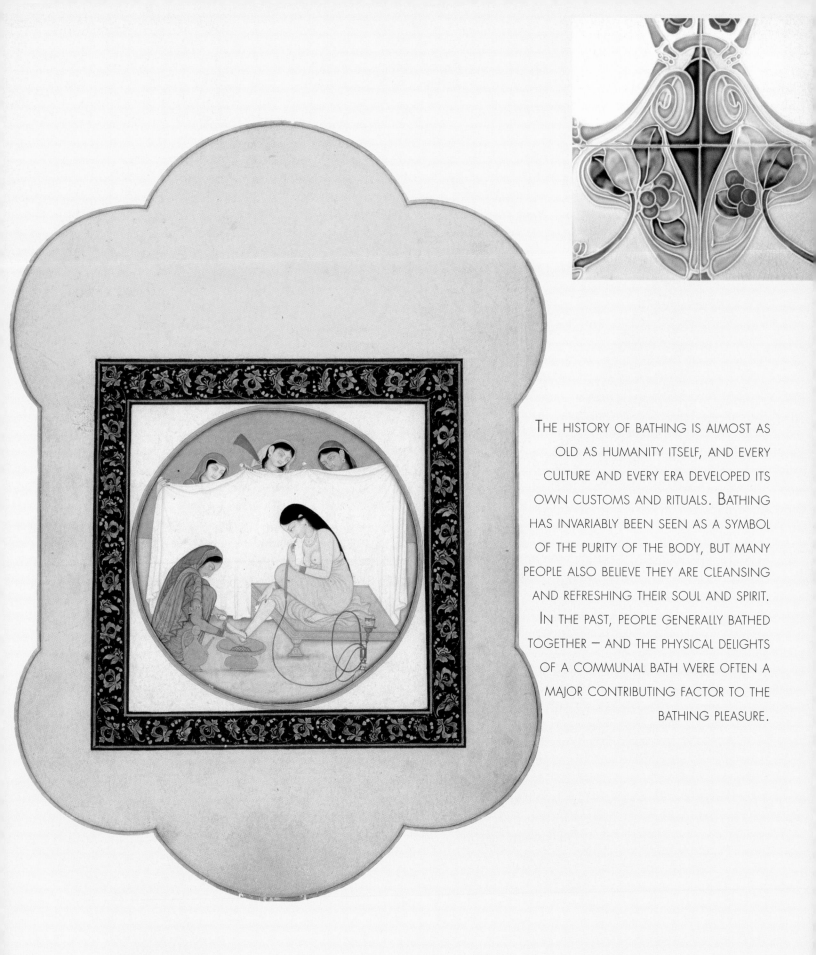

THE HISTORY OF BATHING IS ALMOST AS OLD AS HUMANITY ITSELF, AND EVERY CULTURE AND EVERY ERA DEVELOPED ITS OWN CUSTOMS AND RITUALS. BATHING HAS INVARIABLY BEEN SEEN AS A SYMBOL OF THE PURITY OF THE BODY, BUT MANY PEOPLE ALSO BELIEVE THEY ARE CLEANSING AND REFRESHING THEIR SOUL AND SPIRIT. IN THE PAST, PEOPLE GENERALLY BATHED TOGETHER — AND THE PHYSICAL DELIGHTS OF A COMMUNAL BATH WERE OFTEN A MAJOR CONTRIBUTING FACTOR TO THE BATHING PLEASURE.

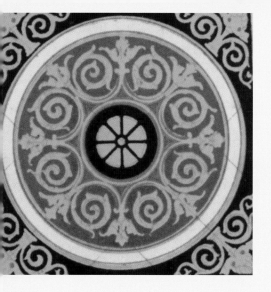
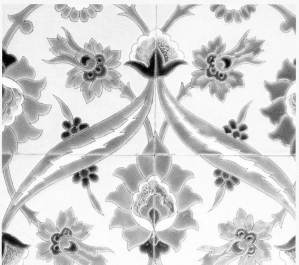
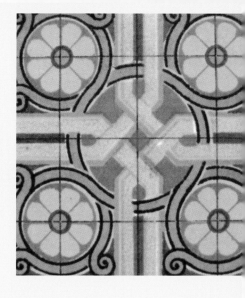

A Brief History
of Bathing Culture

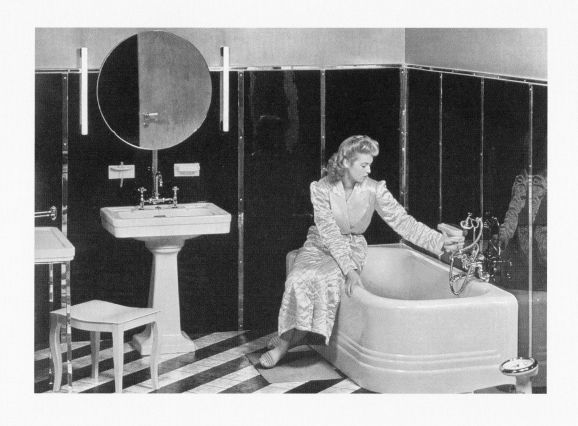

Early Bathing Pleasures

When asked to consider the delights of early historical bathing, most people would immediately think of the Egyptian queen Cleopatra. Her beauty was renowned and she is said to have cared for her skin by spending many hours a day in a bath filled with ass's milk. However, Cleopatra was by no means the first to discover the bliss of bathing. As far back as 4500 BC, Mesopotamian rulers had clay baths installed in their palaces. The large houses in Mahenjo-Daro (in today's Pakistan) were equipped with bathrooms and toilets even back then. The town also had its own pool, although this was reserved for religious ablutions.

Religious ceremonies were accompanied by very strict cleansing rituals. The purifying power of the water for body and soul has been stressed by almost all religious founders – from Buddha to Moses. The oldest reports on record (from around 5000 BC) come from India. There, people were regarded as unclean and untouchable in the morning until they had performed their daily ablutions. Even today, it is fascinating to watch the spectacle of thousands of people bathing in India's sacred rivers.

Religious ablutions have always been and still are a part of all religions: in ancient Egypt, the hands and face had to be washed before one was permitted to pray to Isis. Muslims still have to wash before they are allowed to enter the mosque to pray. In Buddhism, bodily cleanliness is closely connected with spiritual purity and Christian baptism was originally carried out by immersing the entire body in the River Jordan.

However, it would not be correct to put early bathing pleasures exclusively down to religious conscientiousness. Bathing was (and still is) above all synonymous with pleasure, relaxation and bliss.

A good example of this is Greece. The oldest and most famous bathroom (from 1800 BC) can still be viewed in the palace of Knossos on Crete. This room leads on to the queen's chambers and her clay bath is still in quite good condition. Private bathrooms were a privilege of the rich and powerful. The common people, especially the men, met after sport in the shower rooms adjoining the gymnasium. As far back as Homer's time, the Greeks had cultivated bathing to such an extent that day-to-day life would have been unthinkable without it. After sporting competitions, the contestants showered in cold water to steel the body. But people soon discovered that

A Roman bath

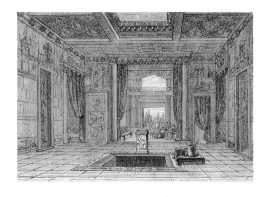

sitting in a bath filled with hot water was much more pleasurable. However, in those days the preference was for public baths that were fitted out with every imaginable comfort, so that these soon became a social meeting place. While the philosophers of ancient Greece protested loudly at what they described as the "effemination" of morals, they had to bow to public pressure in the end. After discovering the delights of hot water, the Greeks went on to investigate the pleasures of steam baths followed by a relaxing massage. They did all this to care for their bodies and comply with the contemporary ideals of beauty.

These social get-togethers in a relaxing atmosphere also pleased the Romans. At first, they only bathed in cool streams and lakes. They also believed that cold water was the essence of physical health; bathing in icy cold water demanded strict discipline and separated the "real men" from the boys. Inspired by the Greeks, rich Romans opened bathing houses, so-called "balneae", where visitors were charged an entrance fee. There they discovered the blessings of warm baths and the strengthening properties of alternating hot and cold baths. A new era began in 19 BC, when General Marcus Vipsanius Agrippa had a superlative bathhouse built (with its own park and artificial lake). He called it his "thermae" (from the Greek "thermos" meaning hot). Unlike the Greeks, however, the Romans were not concerned in the least with physical training – they visited the thermal baths to maintain their good health and cleanliness. The main reason for a visit to the baths, however, was simply to have a good time and enjoy oneself. Before long, luxurious bathhouses began to spring up everywhere. The Romans soon learned to perfect this and they created the first bath landscapes with pools and gardens, steam bath-like sweat rooms and zones of tranquillity. There were sport and play areas, restaurants and theatres. The Roman bathing culture experienced its heyday under the rule of Emperor Nero.

These bathing facilities were enormous – up to 3,000 square metres (30,000 square feet), with separate entrances for men and women. However, to ensure that the two sexes did in fact meet, they installed a sophisticated system of passageways. According to contemporary reports, there was a real carnival atmosphere in the thermae. Music was played, and food and beverages were served in abundance; merchants plied their wares, transactions were made and contracts signed.

As the bathing facilities were now open to all Roman citizens free of charge and were used equally by men and women of every social class, they

All religions had ritual ablution baths. For instance, the "mikwe" was very important in the Jewish religion. The Talmud instructed all believers to "avoid cities that had no public baths."

The native Americans, the Indians, met in "bathing huts" to enjoy a communal steam bath. Cold water was poured over heated stones in the middle of the hut to produce the steam.

The Greeks bathed once a day, often for several hours, in the afternoon before the evening meal. Their cleansing rituals served the aim of achieving the perfect body. The social aspect was merely a positive side-effect.

soon became the subject of much critical discussion. The main criticism was levelled at the lax moral attitude: men and women together in the bath, and not only that, but naked... Christianity soon spoke out against the baths – it condemned nakedness and described the baths as a cesspool of iniquity.

In AD 320, the Council of Laodicea forbade women from entering the baths. This was followed at the end of the 4th century by a general ban.

The thermae that had been opened in other Roman provinces did not last for long after the Fall of the Roman Empire. Under the influence of the Catholic Church, they were closed one after the other.

While the Romans had perfected bathing to a fine art, the Celts and Germanic peoples were rather more rustic in their bathing habits. They also preferred sitting in their bathhouses and sweating together to bathing in private. Cleansing rituals were intended to strengthen clan bonds, but of course, communal bathing was also a great pleasure.

BATHING IN THE MIDDLE AGES – SENSUAL PLEASURES

The Church only put a temporary stop to the opulent pleasures of bathing by instilling a sense of chasteness in the people. While the monks continued to bathe in the monasteries as before, the common folk were deprived of this pleasure. However, in spite of all reserves, in the Middle Ages there developed a new type of bathing culture that quickly spread throughout the whole of Europe. The bathing customs were "new" in the sense that new dimensions were opened up through the experiences that the Crusaders had collected during their military campaigns. For instance, the Oriental "hammam" steam bath had a particular influence on the bathing customs of those days. Admittedly, in Europe the people were not quite so demure as in the Orient. There, the baths were strictly separated according to sex, whereas in Europe people were not quite so fussy. The Europeans enjoyed being pampered while taking a long hot bath: the bath maids and servants were not just concerned with body care, they also offered their services as prostitutes and procurers. They were renowned for their special massages and were therefore also known as "rubbers".

Man and woman in a bath, woodcut from 1481

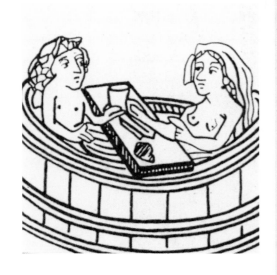

Page opposite: The singer Jakob von der Warte bathing in a garden, 14th century

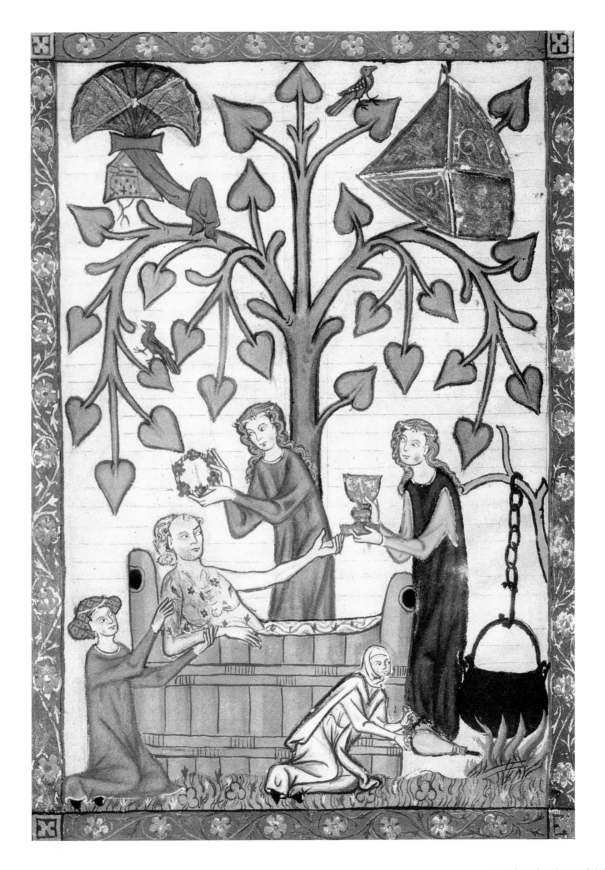

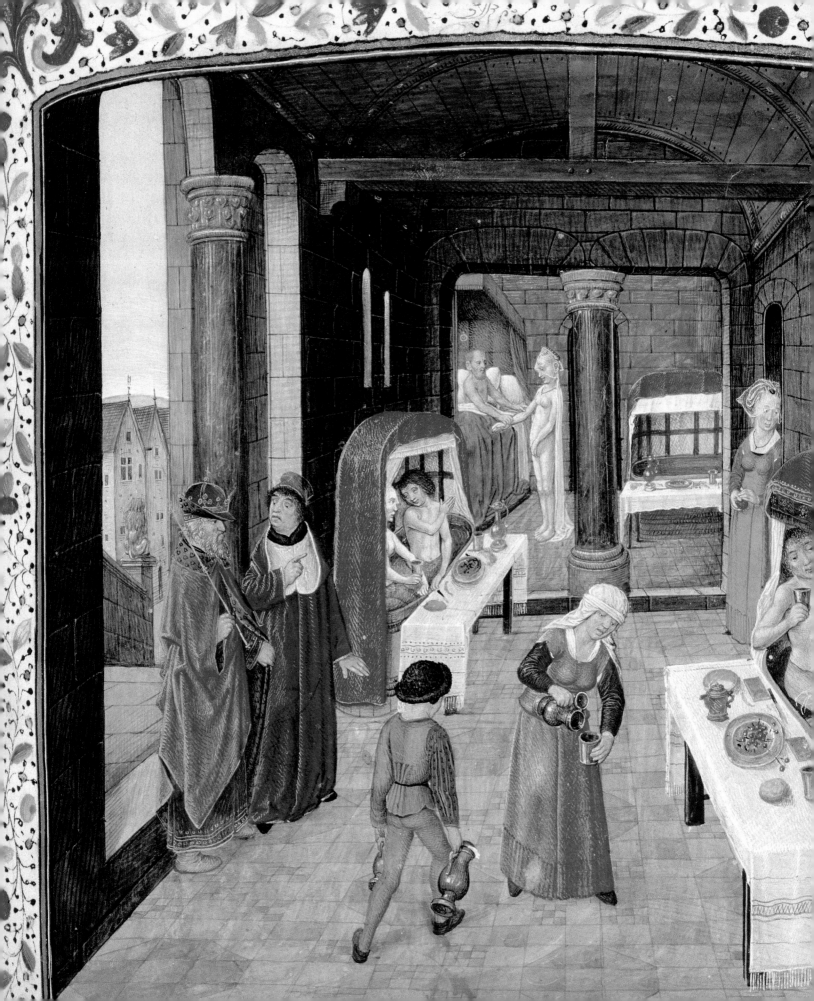

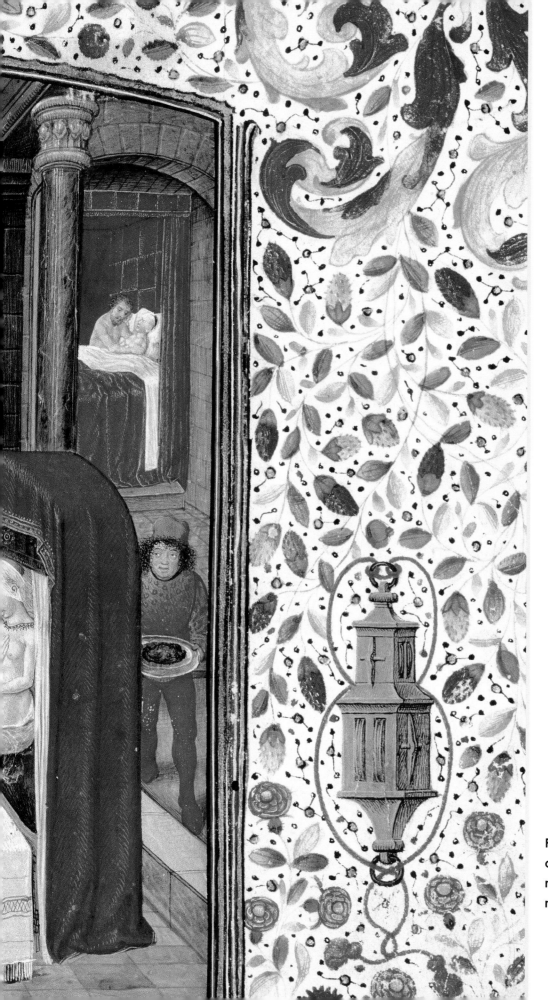

Public baths, Master from the court
of Duke Antoine of Burgundy,
miniature from the Valerius Maximus
manuscript, c. 1470

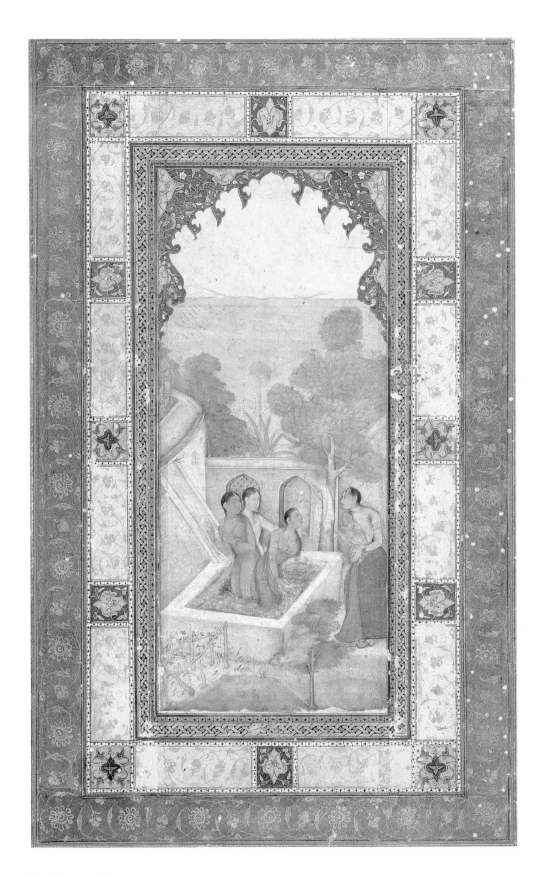

Agnes Bernauer was a celebrated bath maid who fell in love with Duke Albrecht of Bavaria in 1432. However, their secret wedding did not bring her much luck: her father-in-law denounced her as a witch and had her drowned in the Danube in 1435.

It might seem a little shocking that books and articles were written about the easy-going morals in the public baths, and that in all openness. One example of this is the "Romance of the Rose" by French author G. de Lorris, who wrote, "The young men and women who have been rounded up by the old procuresses go there; they roam through the meadows and fruit groves as happy as parrots and then they go together to the bathing chambers and bathe together in the same bath…"

This new-found freedom went along well with the latest medical findings, which the Persian doctor and philosopher Ibn Sina had compiled in his work *Canon medicinae*. He had clearly recognised the importance of physical toughening and hygiene for body and soul alike. Alternating hot and cold baths, massage and gymnastics experienced a real renaissance.

In the 13th and 14th centuries, running a bathhouse was regarded as a respectable profession. Anyone who could afford the entrance fee was permitted to enter and could then relax in hot baths and languorous steam baths, dine on sumptuous banquets and lounge in exquisite relaxation zones. New professions were established: the bathing attendant, the beard shaver and the wound doctor. Besides shaving, body depilation and hair-cuts, health cures were offered in the bathhouses, in the form of treatment with leeches, massages and blood-letting.

However, by this time the people had also begun bathing zealously at home. Although they only possessed simple wooden tubs which they filled with hot water, they soon learned the benefits of adding healing herbs that made every bath a pleasure. Even war-weary generals enjoyed climbing into the bath after a day on the battlefield.

Over the centuries, the comforts of private bathrooms became more and more sophisticated. The wooden tub was gradually replaced by a more elegant model in zinc or silver. At the same time, heating techniques were improved and small boilers that were used to heat the water were directly connected to the bath. Bathrooms and pavilions were erected, and in the stately homes the first pipes were laid for running hot and cold water.

Page opposite: Ladies bathing, album leaflet from the Akbar period, c. 1590

Those who could afford such private bathing pleasures were much more concerned with the fun factor than with the hygiene that went along with it. European rulers competed with one another to create more beautiful and more unusual bathing refuges. And the clergy were no less active in this quest.

Against the background of these developments and the general pleasure derived from bathing, it is somewhat difficult to comprehend why the bathing era came to an end in the way it did. Although there were some faint-hearted attempts to speak out against the decline of the bathing era (by Montaigne, for example), these were in vain. The age of "dry hygiene" had begun.

A Bathing Intermission: Two Centuries of Dry Hygiene

Within the space of only a few decades, bathing culture in 16th-century Europe had lost a tremendous amount of its popularity. There appear to be no specific historical reasons for this; however, several individual factors were probably decisive. On the one hand, there was a general change of attitude: while up until this time everything "physical" had been accepted as nature-given, there was now an increasing feeling of modesty in matters of the body; this was reflected in a particular repression in the area of hygiene.

Bathhouse and brothel came to be increasingly regarded as one and the same thing. Such licentious pleasure was condemned, and many bathhouses finally had to close their doors once and for all.

On the other hand, the Plague was spreading at an alarming rate, taking along more and more victims in its path. The bathhouses were said to be partly responsible for the spread of this pandemic.

And on top of this, the circumstances of the people of those days had changed drastically. Wars flaring up all over the place took their toll, and the Plague could not be contained. As a result, fewer and fewer people were able to find joy in the lightheartedness of pleasurable bathing. Life had become harder and the joie de vivre of former times suffered accordingly. Apparently however, no one considered that by condemning bathing they were also condemning cleanliness.

The widespread permissiveness in many baths was the cause of their demise shortly afterwards. Criticism from the Church became increasingly severe and the spread of the Plague and syphilis did the rest to put an end to the pleasures of bathing.

Nowadays, on looking back it seems almost grotesque that in the 18th century, a time when bathing culture was literally at rock bottom, the fine arts such as music and literature were experiencing an upswing like never before – or since.

The Reformation and Counter-Reformation also ensured that nakedness was condemned as a sin and that everything physical was seen as unclean.

And over the course of the years, this dirt became accepted as a fact of life. Concealing all the filth with white shirts and underwear was in no way successful. Lavishly powdered wigs and starched collars could only conceal the lack of personal hygiene on the surface. Still, white underwear was regarded as a synonym for a "clean" mind. This made it particularly easy for the ruling classes to regard the poor and often dirty vassals as a depraved rabble. A person who was not in a position to care for his or her outward appearance was thought not to have impeccable morals.

When people washed themselves, it was done very much in private, and they usually limited themselves to washing just their face and hands. The many steam baths that had once abounded in Paris had been reduced to just two by the reign of Louis XIV; and these specialised exclusively in medically prescribed therapeutic baths.

The water even began to run dry in private bathrooms. The anti-bathing front was given medical support. Doctor Louis Savot wrote in 1624, "We can do without bathing much better than our forefathers because we use underwear that helps us keep our body clean in a more comfortable fashion than the baths and steam baths used by our forebears, who knew nothing of the use or comfort of this underwear." And by way of confirmation, they blamed water for all the evils of this world. It was said to weaken the body and cause toxic transpiration as well as promote imbecility and dropsy.

So-called "dry hygiene" was carried out as follows: only the hands and mouth were given some superficial care. The hair was shampooed dry and rapidly hidden under a

Jug from a washing set of Emperor Wilhelm I.

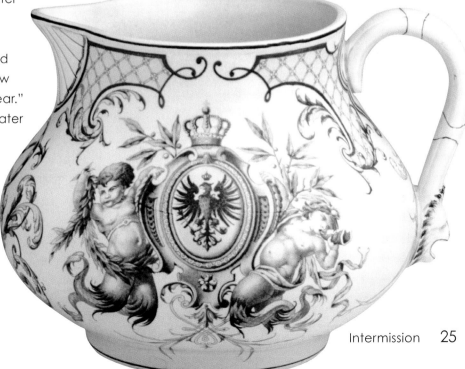

wig. Colourful makeup and perfumed powder replaced facial hygiene; people poured perfume over themselves and placed fragrant smelling sachets under their arms. Contact with water was very sparing and only took place behind closed doors.

In sharp contrast to all of this, new, increasingly elegant bathrooms were being installed in the palaces. But the sumptuous baths enormous size, more and more sophisticated technology in the preparation of hot water and artistically designed tiles on the floors and walls could not disguise the fact that most of these rooms remained unused.

In 1715 the Sun King died, and with his passing the era of dry hygiene also came to an end.

The 18th Century: A Renaissance of Bathing Culture

This rediscovery of naturalness was promoted in Europe by the philosophers of the Enlightenment: Rousseau, Voltaire and Diderot in France, Locke in England and Basedow in Germany. They were supported by the medical profession, which testified to the health-promoting effects of regular alternating hot and cold baths. Lavoisier's discovery in 1777 that the skin breathes was nothing short of revolutionary.

From now on it was acceptable to bathe again, and the people did it with pleasure. Luxurious bathrooms were soon being installed in the palaces of the ruling classes and in the villas of the rich and famous. Although the situation was by no means encouraging in the public bath domain, more comfortable baths were developed that compensated for this to a certain extent. For some time, portable models were in vogue and these proved highly popular even with the lower social classes. In houses with no room for a separate bathroom, one had to be flexible. In many cases, the baths were simply set up in the kitchen whenever needed, because the hot water was close by. In the 19th century, running water was still a privilege of wealthy citizens.

Mobile bathtubs were placed either in the kitchen or in the hallway. After all, every single bucket of water had to be carried to the tub – and the shortest path was the most practical.

Art nouveau ornamentation on mural tiles

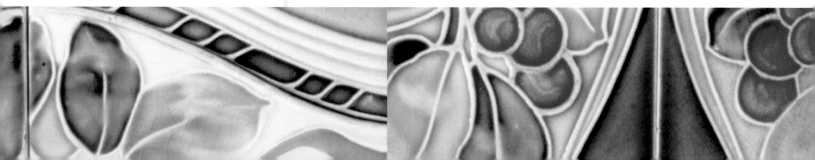

Despite these unfavourable conditions, great emphasis was now placed on bathing in general and on hygiene in particular. Medical research was making rapid advances and was able to demonstrate a definite connection between hygiene and health. The beneficial effects of water were rediscovered and propagated by men such as Hufland, Priessnitz, Rikli and Lassar.

Cleanliness became a moral dictate and many books were written at this time that were concerned with the importance of bathing. However, these demands were virtually impossible to fulfil, since the prerequisites were simply not in place.

Throughout Europe those who were not quite so wealthy were assisted in their quest for hygiene by the opening of "public baths". "Family hygiene" was preached with almost prophetic zeal. But in the urban centres, there was hardly any running water – not to mention the situation in rural areas. Besides this, the disposal of the waste water posed somewhat of a problem. It was expensive to heat the water and thus the idea of installing private bathrooms throughout the country was out of the question.

Public baths were opened for children, communal showers were set up for industrial workers and the rural communities themselves in the rivers. Around 1855, an idea came from France of combining the public baths and laundry facilities in the one institution. The first of these in Germany was opened in Hamburg, where 75 baths and laundry facilities with running hot water were installed. Later, these were perfected even further to comprise baths and showers in first and second-class versions. This was a step in the wrong direction: the simple folk were soon no longer able to afford the use of these establishments. Towards the end of the 19th century, the public baths were being replaced to an increasing extent by showers, which were soon nicknamed "the common people's bath".

Private bathrooms for everyone were an illusion that was not particularly easy to put into practice. The following quotation from a "national education treatise" clearly illustrates just how "neglected" the bathing culture had become by this time. The French teacher Massé wrote in 1845:

Difficult as it was to convince the common folk to care for their personal hygiene, the rich enjoyed the luxury of a bath all the more. In Paris a new fashion was established – the "bathing cabinet". In well-to-do households, this intimate washroom was found next to the bedroom.

Even the ancient Greeks showered. In the 19th century, the shower experienced a renaissance as the "common people's bath".

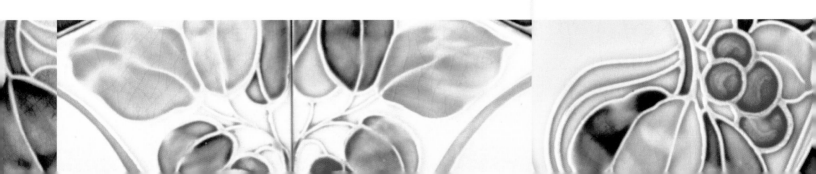

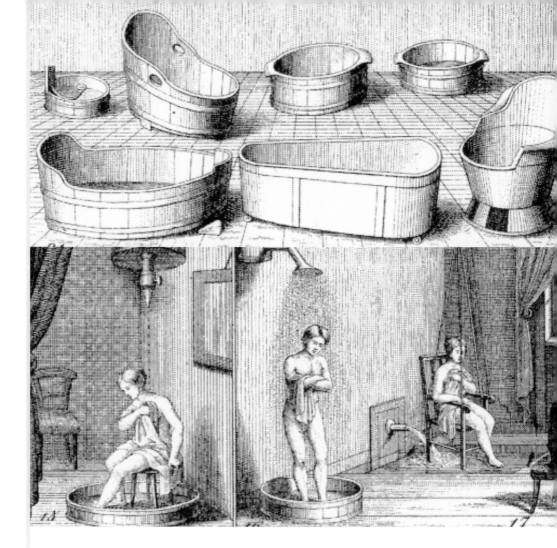

Top: Bathing and sitting tubs and washing vessels from the 19th century
Left: Brip bath; centre: Shower bath; right: Device for lowering the infirm into a bath, all 19th century

"A basin half full of cold water, a small kettle filled with hot water, two large sponges…, a large piece of flannel, and towels or face cloths. Take a woollen cloth and rub the whole body with it. Especially rub the chest, the armpits and all parts where the warmth of the bed could have caused perspiration… Now, take the two sponges, one in each hand, dip them in the basin and begin washing resolutely…"

A BATHROOM OF ONE'S OWN: LUXURY (NOT) FOR EVERYONE

Up to the end of the 19th century, a private bathroom remained a luxury that only very few wealthy people could afford. It was very rare to find a bathroom firmly installed in a house or even just a room set aside for the purpose of bathing. This lack of facilities was a golden opportunity for the inventors of mobile shower cabinets and cupboard baths, which could also be set up in the hallway. Soon some of the models even went into mass production.

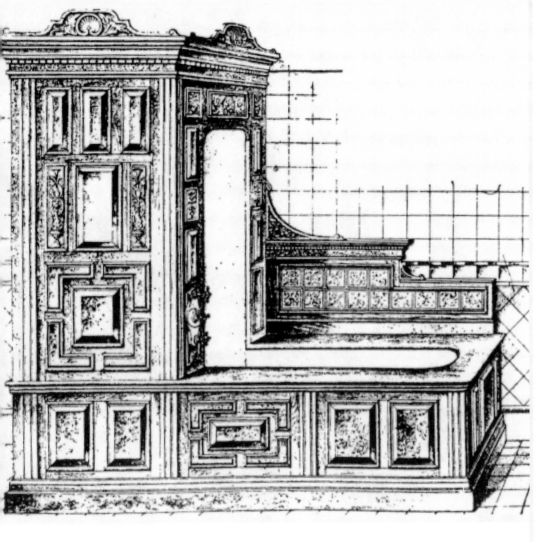

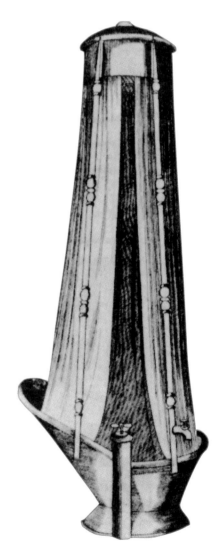

Left: Bath with "hood", England, late 19th century
Below: Sitting bath with shower, England, mid-19th century

The real revolution in the bathroom eventually came from America. At a hygiene exhibition in 1900, visitors were able to see and admire an American bathroom for the first time. At the beginning of the 20th century, bathrooms were beginning to be incorporated into in house plans. A number of technological innovations had led to the rise of a new bathing culture and, at the same time, an unprecedented level of hygiene-consciousness. Ease of cleaning the bathroom took priority over aesthetic trappings. Vicious tongues referred to this type of design as the "dirt removal machine", and in actual fact the US model was more reminiscent of a sterile laboratory than a comfortable, aesthetically pleasing bathroom. The soft mats were replaced by bare tiles – bacteria were to be given no mercy whatsoever. However, the new trend corresponded to the zeitgeist, according to which hygiene had top priority.

The dream of a bathroom of one's own became generally known as the "American bath". This had a standard design, consisting of a large bath, a basin and a toilet. The room was functional and absolutely hygienic. There was no room for imaginative design here. This became the pattern for the

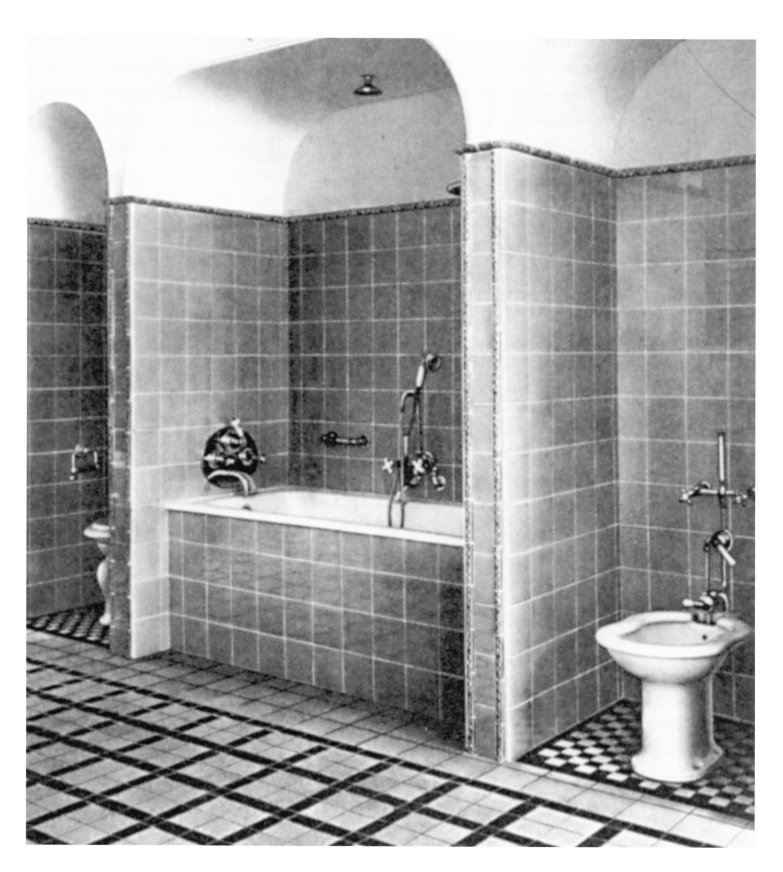

bathrooms that were later to be built in housing estates throughout Germany after World War II.

In the years between the World Wars, Germany was still largely lacking a genuine bathing culture. The trend was more towards "wet cells" which allowed not much more than rudimentary hygiene. However, this was the principal aim in any case; after all, bathing was not supposed to be pleasurable – it was a necessary evil, a hygienic measure for keeping the body healthy.

From then on, developments in private bathrooms accelerated at breakneck speed, and practicality was the number one priority. Around the middle of the 1960s, the sobriety that had been connected with bathing and bathrooms in Europe gradually began to make way for pleasure and aesthetic appeal.

Considering the strict hygiene-consciousness and the prudery of the time, what a sensation it must have been in 1954 when Marilyn Monroe could be seen lounging in a foam-filled bath in the film *The Seven Year Itch*! We can probably thank the film stars of that age and the initiative of countless magazines for the rediscovery of bathing for pleasure.

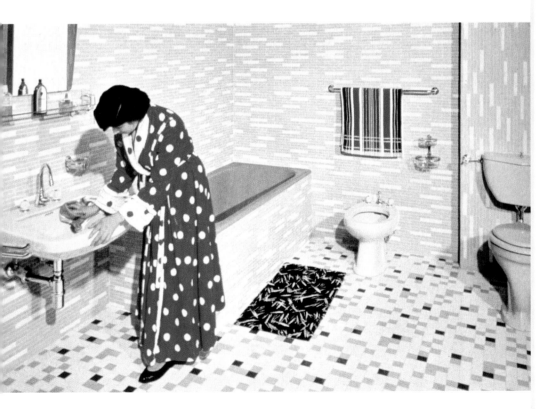

Page opposite: Bathroom from the period between the World Wars
Left: Bathroom from the time of the German 'economic miracle'

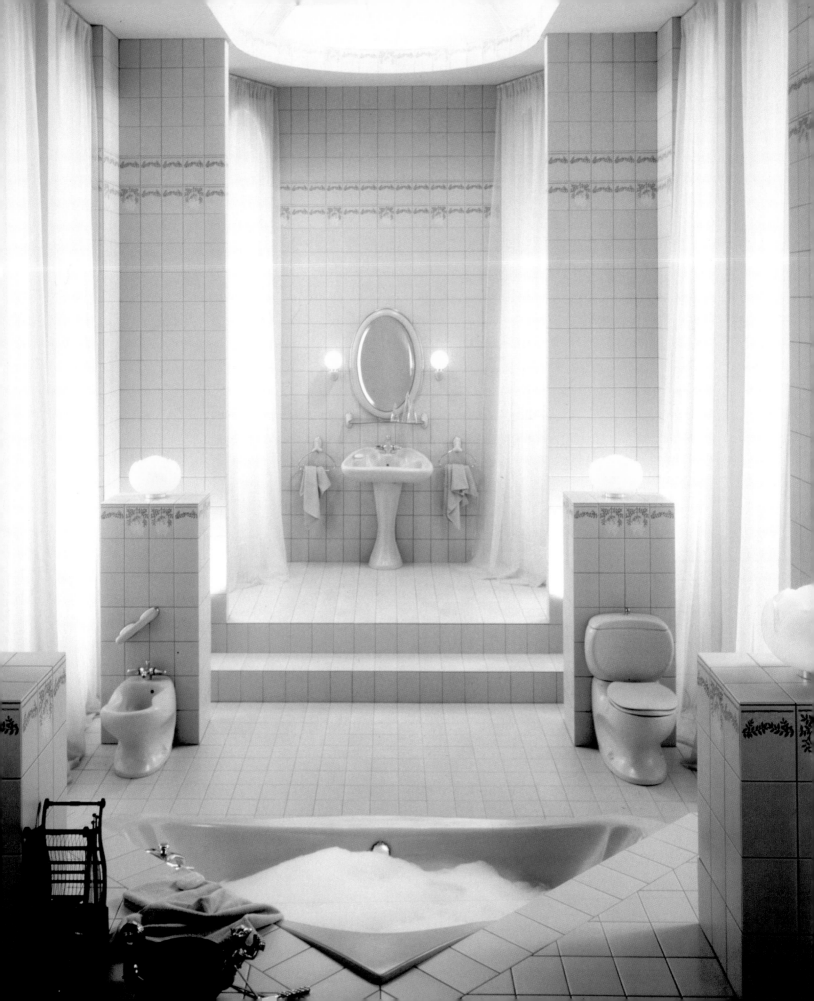

In the meantime, bathroom technology and design have advanced much further; and today there is virtually no one devoid of bathing facilities in the western world. The morning shower is a treasured ritual and the evening bath a pleasure. However, looking back, it can be said that the true hey-day of bathing lies almost two thousand years in the past.

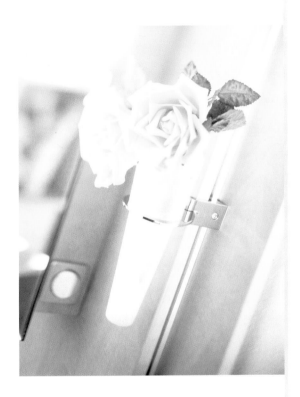

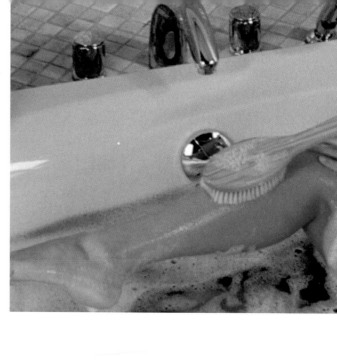

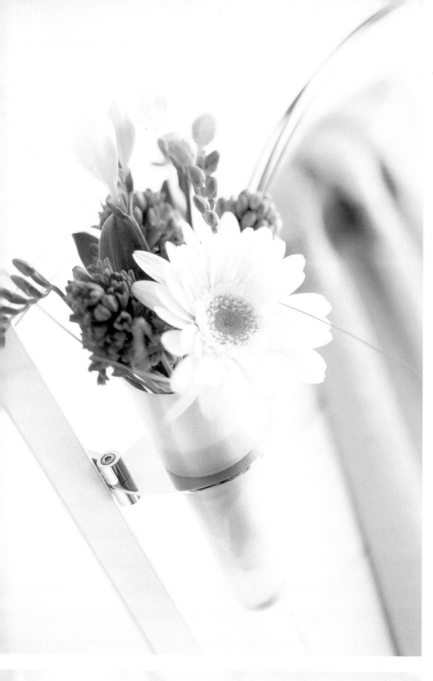

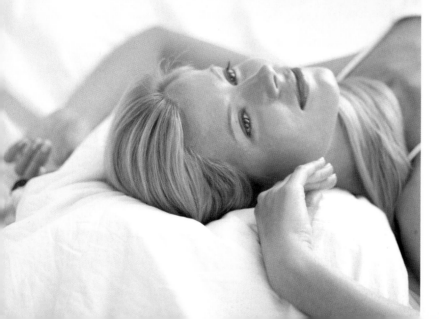

Simply switch off, rinse off your stress and fill up with new energy — everyone needs to do this now and then. Just forget the world with all its hustle and bustle and step in — you can do this best at home in your own bathroom. Even the murmuring of the water as it runs into the bathtub awakens pleasant associations: the refreshing babbling of a mountain brook, the roar of the waves as they roll onto the sand at the beach, the lashing of the foam as the surf thunders towards the rocks. The anticipation is surpassed only by your actual experience of the pleasure of the bath. The cosy feeling of a hot bathtub after a long winter's walk, the tingling refreshment of a cool shower after a hot summer's day — water, a seemingly so simple element, offers pure relaxation for body and soul.

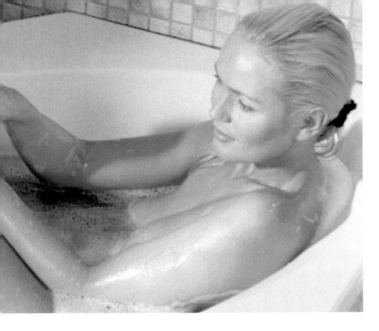

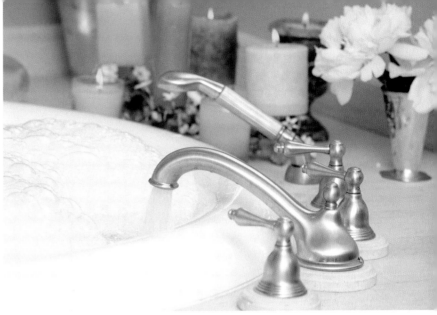

Bath Essentials

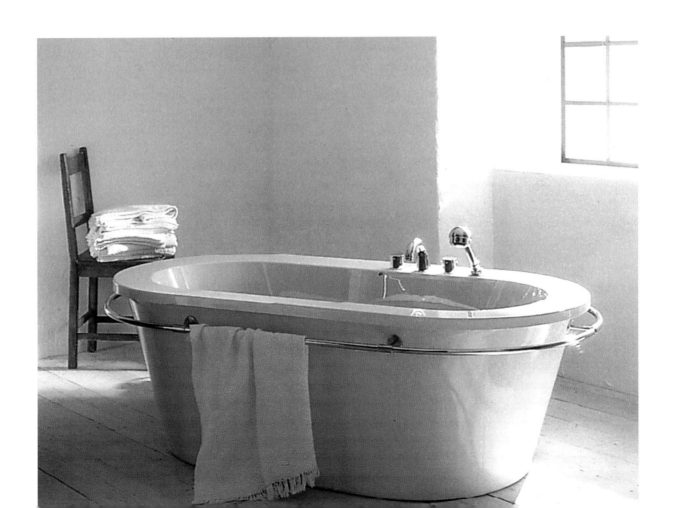

THE BATH IS MORE THAN A SENSUOUS WATERY PLEASURE

A bath is the simplest way of doing something good for your body. You only really need to fill a tub with water and step in – that is all there is to it. You require no technology and no lavish equipment. On the other hand, a warm bath is extremely effective: it purifies the skin and relaxes the muscles. The warmth dilates the blood vessels and stimulates the circulation. Your metabolism is stimulated to eliminate more harmful substances from your body. And when your mind is relaxed, this also has a calming effect on troubled nerves.

The healing power of the bath is considerably reinforced if certain bath additives are used. Depending on the choice of preparation, you can bring about an improvement to your insomnia or avert a cold that is threatening to develop. A bath is effective in countless ways, and it can work wonders in alleviating both mental problems and physical ailments.

When you consider its multitude of beneficial effects, it becomes clear that a bath affects the organism in its entirety. On the one hand this is good, but it can also be hazardous – after all, anything that has a positive effect on the whole body can also harm it if put to use unwisely. It is therefore important to pay attention to some basic rules when bathing.

Relaxation from the word go – the bathroom is an oasis of peace and recuperation.

TAKE CARE!

When we get into the bathtub, we do not often think much about the consequences of our actions beforehand. However simple and soothing baths may be, not everyone can enjoy all types of bath without encountering some problem or other. People who suffer from cardiovascular disorders should be particularly careful. When taking a bath, a person with high blood pressure is at least as much at risk as someone with blood pressure that is too low. People with heart problems should consult a doctor in any case.

Why this caution? People who have an unstable cardiovascular system are sure to be familiar with the symptoms that come about through sudden

Note the critical "turning point": this occurs at a water temperature of 38–39 °C (100–102 °F), at which the relaxing effect can give way to a stimulating one.

changes in the weather or extreme differences in altitude. In this instance, it is the changes in air pressure that have an effect on the body. Warm baths have a somewhat similar effect: the weight of the water gives rise to so-called hydrostatic pressure that can have an effect similar to changes in air pressure. Possible consequences can be anything from nausea to a circulatory collapse. To aggravate this situation, warm or hot water also stimulates cardiac activity. People with heart disease are therefore better off doing without hot baths unless they consult a doctor.

People suffering from arteriosclerosis must not take alternating baths, because their blood vessels might no longer be versatile enough to cope with the stimulus. Applications with cold water are not suitable for these risk groups.

The precautions for high and low blood pressure are similar: not too long, not too hot and no intensively acting bath additives. It is best to gradually try out which type of bath best fulfils your personal needs. At first, you should not stay in the bath for more than five minutes; you can then gradually extend your bathing time.

Feelings of dizziness and nausea are clear signs that the bath does not agree with you. As soon as you notice this, you should get out of the bath straight away; but do so slowly, and after you have dried yourself you should lie down with your legs propped up.

Hot baths can also cause problems for people who suffer from venous problems, i.e. from varicose veins or pronounced minor varicose dilatations of the cutaneous veins. Baths that are close to body temperature are the best suited for these people. Moreover, they too should only gradually increase the duration of the bath, beginning with five minutes.

People with pronounced couperosis – these are pronounced dilatations of the veins, particularly on the face and neckline – also cannot tolerate hot baths. Those affected should also refrain from going to the sauna.

Of course, pregnancy is not an illness, but women should be careful during this very special time. Baths that are too hot and contain stimulating bath additives can cause problems. On the

The Most Important Bathing Rules

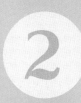

Tired? Off to Bed and Not into the Tub!

If you are feeling tired and completely washed out, you should not be taking a bath. Tiredness of this kind tends to indicate cardiovascular weakness or the beginning of an infection. In such cases, a bath is out of the question. On the other hand, if you are only slightly tired, a bath may well refresh you.

To Feel Totally Well – Plan in Advance

A suitable ambience increases your feeling of well-being. A portable radio or a CD player can provide relaxing music. The music intensifies relaxation and makes way for pleasant feelings and thoughts. Avoid getting out of the tub while bathing; the body could lose heat and so the bath may not have the desired effect.

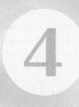

It Should be Pleasantly Warm

For a relaxing bath, the surrounding room temperature must be suitably matched to that of the water. The best temperature for getting undressed – and later for getting out of the bath without shivering – is 20–30 °C (68–86 °F). If you want an even greater feeling of well-being with fragrant oils, you can set up an aroma lamp (but for safety reasons, at a safe distance from the bath!).

Comfort and Luxury are no Mere Trickery

If you want to thoroughly spoil yourself, you will need to make a few preparations and use some equipment. A head cushion attached to the edge of the bath with suckers is a useful accessory for the tub. To avoid the risk of slipping, you should place a warm slip-protection mat on the floor next to the bath. And to avoid excessive cooling, which would be therapeutically undesirable, you should wrap yourself in pre-warmed bath towels as soon as you step out.

No Food – no Alcohol

An integral part of any program of spoiling yourself in the bath is most definitely a glass of champagne. Mind you, one should be very careful about drinking alcohol when taking a bath, and it can also be dangerous to handle glasses in the bathroom. Incidentally, grandma's bath rule "don't eat before bathing" still applies today.

Pay Attention to the Colour of your Face!

The colour of your face gives an important indication of whether the bath is also doing you good. A paler facial teint than usual could indicate low blood pressure. The same applies if a cold sweat should develop. The opposite too (an extremely red face) is a warning: it indicates a build-up of heat. In both cases you should terminate your bath.

The Time of Day Makes a Difference

Our body temperature changes somewhat over the course of the day. The organism really heats up between about 3 a.m. and 3 p.m. The feeling of coldness in the limbs increases with rising body temperature. If you bathe at these times, you should not finish off with a cold shower. Incidentally, the sauna effect is the best at this time of day, and cold treatments are less unpleasant.

Goose Pimples? Your Body is Reacting Wrongly!

Anyone who shivers during a cool or warm bath or who develops goose pimples should get out of the bath. An excessive pulse rate also shows that the body is reacting wrongly.

Height, Weight, Sex – Calculate Correctly!

The taller and heavier a person is, the less heat the body absorbs. When people of differing physical build share a bath, the temperature must be chosen to suit both. You should not have too hot a bath if a child is with you. The ideal temperature can also deviate in the case of elderly people and children, and must be selected individually. However, there are hardly any differences regarding sex, except that women are more sensitive to heat before menstruation and react more intensely to cold.

Before Bathing – Measure your Blood Pressure

If your blood pressure generally tends to be either quite high or very low, you should measure it before taking a bath. Furthermore, make sure your feet are warm, and soap down your body so that sebaceous matter does not prevent the penetration of beneficial active substances.

Never Carry out Bath Therapy Alone

If you would like to relax with an intensive therapy bath, you will need to be particularly careful. As you can never precisely predict the body's re-action, you should not be alone. It is best to agree on a signal you can give to alert someone. Then slip into a warm bed for your nightly rest and drink another two glasses of still mineral water before going to sleep.

6

7

8

9

10

11

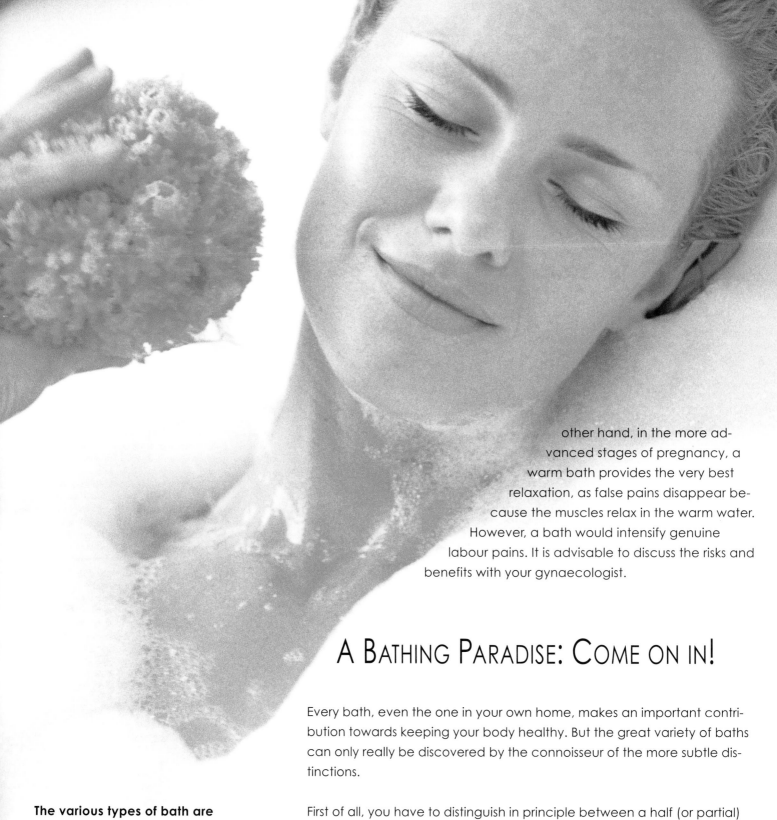

other hand, in the more advanced stages of pregnancy, a warm bath provides the very best relaxation, as false pains disappear because the muscles relax in the warm water. However, a bath would intensify genuine labour pains. It is advisable to discuss the risks and benefits with your gynaecologist.

A Bathing Paradise: Come on in!

Every bath, even the one in your own home, makes an important contribution towards keeping your body healthy. But the great variety of baths can only really be discovered by the connoisseur of the more subtle distinctions.

The various types of bath are distinguished by the amount of water used and the temperature – a bath thermometer is thus indispensable.

First of all, you have to distinguish in principle between a half (or partial) and a full bath. As the name already implies, in the one type the tub is only half full and in the other it is completely full. Expressed in figures, for a partial or half bath you need about 100 to 150 litres (25 to 40 gallons), and for a full bath, depending on the design of the bath, you need 200 to 300 litres

(50 to 75 gallons). A further distinction is made with regard to the different temperatures. So you can talk about a hot bath, a cold bath, a rising temperature bath and a poikilothermic bath.

THE HOT BATH

In the case of a hot bath, heat is supplied to the body – this enhances the production of perspiration. The metabolism is stimulated, so that increased amounts of harmful substances can be eliminated. The blood vessels and muscles relax in the cosy warmth so that the blood pressure is reduced and you feel pleasantly sleepy. These effects can be achieved at a bath temperature of around 38 °C (100 °F), and you should stay in the bath for about 15 to 20 minutes.

THE COLD BATH

A cold bath is only suitable if the body is well warmed through. The sensation of cold stimulates the metabolism, the cardiovascular system, the nervous system and the body's own defences. Cold baths require a water temperature of about 12–15 °C (54–60 °F) and should not last longer than 5 to 25 seconds.

THE RISING TEMPERATURE BATH

This bath really gets your body moving: the temperature is initially about 35 °C (95 °F) and is increased over the space of ten minutes to 39–41 °C (102–106 °F) by running hot water into it. The effect is sudorific and antispasmodic; however, 15 to 20 minutes are sufficient. The correct time to get out is when you break out in sweat. Then you should have a cool shower and rest up in bed for half an hour.

THE POIKILOTHERMIC BATH

This type of bath increases the body's defences and is a good exercise for the blood vessels. It is rather difficult to make a full or half bath poikilothermic because most people only own one tub; you can just as well sit in the bath and then get under the shower. The bath temperature is around 37 °C

Bathing properly also means heeding the reactions of your own body and acting accordingly.

(99 °F) and you bathe in it for 3 to 5 minutes. Then you alternate and have a cold shower for 10 to 20 seconds; you then get back in the bath. You should alternate three times in all.

THE HOT BATH

The hot bath is an exception, since it is essentially taken for chronic colds and as a therapeutic treatment. Its temperature ranges from 38 to 40 °C (100 to 104 °F) and its duration from 10 to 60 minutes. Typical indications are gout and arthritis, and this type of bath is also used in cosmetic therapy for the treatment of cellulitis. As such long hot baths are not tolerated well by everyone, you should not take them if you are alone in the house. It is better if another person is close by so that help is at hand in an emergency.

SINK INTO A MOUNTAIN OF FOAM

When it comes to well-being, the foam bath is the "classic". As soon as you look at it, you feel like sinking into its fantastic foam, but foam baths are generally not ideal for the skin. The surfactants contained in them take the oil out of the skin and dry it out.

These days, there are also products that include "re-oiling additives" so as to prevent precisely this from occurring. However, this skin-sparing variant mostly comes at the cost of the foam, which can then only form in moderation – these are the so-called cream foam baths.

If you really want to have the most voluminous foam bath possible, you will have to prepare it well. For this you put 15 to 20 ml ($^1/_2$ to $^2/_3$ oz) of bath additives in the empty tub and make this really froth up with the water from the shower nozzle. The more stable the foam, the better the water temperature under it will remain.

BATHING WITH A BONUS FOR YOUR HEALTH

Water itself is of course quite beneficial on its own, but in combination with healing bath additives its effects are greatly intensified. The more natural these additives are, the greater the benefit to be expected. Several examples show this clearly.

When you take a foam bath, you do not need additional soap – this would only cause the foam to collapse quickly. It is important to have a shower to remove all foam residue before getting out of the bath.

Spa baths are particularly pleasant. With a simple spa bath mat, you can transform your own tub into a massage pool in next to no time. The agreeable effect is certainly familiar to many who have had an underwater massage, in which the body is treated at a number of individual points. With a spa bath, on the other hand, the pressure of the water is evenly distributed over the entire body via thermo-mechanical skin stimulation. The effect is dramatic: spa baths stimulate the circulation, have a positive influence on the vegetative nervous system, improve breathing and promote healing after injury. They also have cosmetic benefits: spa baths have a peeling effect, make the skin smooth and train the muscles.

You should avoid spa baths if you have problems with your cardiovascular system, suffer from high blood pressure or a high pulse rate; this also applies to inflammatory skin diseases, during pregnancy and if you have a tendency towards varicose veins and other venous disorders.

The Triumphal Advance of Thalassotherapy

The sea is a bounteous, practically inexhaustible source of goodness; it also provides us with bathing water of a very special kind. A litre of sea water contains 35 g of dissolved salts (corresponding to over half an ounce per pint); these comprise all the trace elements, minerals and salt compounds important for the human body – in just the right combination, too.

From the riches of the ocean came sea medicine, also known as thalassotherapy.

The first seaside resort was established in 1730 at Scarborough on the North Sea. As early as 1843 there were thirty in England in the region of the Channel, nineteen on the Atlantic Coast and a further eighteen seaside resorts in the North Sea area. Ireland and Scotland each also had ten seaside resorts. The French Encyclopaedia of Seaside Resorts for Europe already listed no less than eighty such venues in France in 1865.

Thalassotherapy was applied primarily as a treatment for rheumatic diseases, problems of the musculoskeletal system and skin diseases. These days, you no longer have to travel to the ocean to enjoy the healing powers of the sea. Cutting-edge production technologies have made it possible, you might say, to bring the sea to your home through high-quality concentrated products. So now the whole year through you can treat

Caution with sea products is only necessary if you have a thyroid function disorder or are allergic to iodine.

Temperatures for Seaweed Sea Baths

Temperature	Effect
25–30 °C (77–86 °F); lukewarm	tones up and stimulates
31–34 °C (88–93 °F); warm	calming and settling
35–36 °C (94–97 °F); warm–hot	relaxing, but only for healthy people
37–38 °C (98–100 °F); hot	helps with weight reduction and against cellulitis (take care if you have heart problems!)

yourself comfortably at home with a whole range of sea products: sea salt, plankton, seaweed, ocean sediment, mud and silt.

When used internally and externally, the home thalasso treatment constitutes a full therapy, the only limitation being that people who are allergic to iodine or who have a thyroid disorder must switch to marine products that do not contain iodine.

Treatment using the thalasso method is generally appropriate in cases of exhaustion, following operations and accidents, for fitness in sport, for coping with stress – for recovery and recuperation in the widest sense of the words. However, astounding results can also be achieved in the case of diseases of the respiratory tracts such as inflammation of the paranasal sinuses, bronchitis, rhinolaryngitis and bronchial asthma. It is also used successfully with skin disorders like acne, couperosis, wrinkles and premature aging of the skin as well as in combating cellulitis, overweight and gynaecological complaints.

Thalasso home baths should be used as a cure two to three times a week. The therapy begins with a bath lasting just five minutes; the time can then be gradually extended to 20 minutes.

Essential Oils: Bathe in Fragrance!

Lean back and relax; just think of the refreshing fragrance of a freshly mown meadow. Shut your eyes and enjoy the aroma of freshly ground coffee.

Our sense of smell is often under-estimated. However, scents often have a major influence on our moods and feelings, even if we are only rarely conscious of this fact.

Essential Oils – A Small Selection

Essential oil	Applications (examples)
Angelica root	strengthens the immune system
Aniseed	stomach, digestion
Basil	intestinal infections, depression, spasms
Bergamot	anxiety, depression
Cardamom	headaches, heartburn
Cinnamon	colds, tension
Eucalyptus	asthma, hay fever, coughs, migraine
Fennel	bronchitis, digestion
Geranium	acne, eczema, wounds, menstrual problems
Jasmine	aphrodisiac, pre-menstrual syndrome
Juniper	skin problems, cellulitis, lumbago
Lavender	acne, skin problems, muscular strain
Lemon	cardiovascular disorders, tension
Lemon balm	headaches, stress, menopause
Marjoram	menstrual problems
Mint	colds, stomach and intestinal problems, migraine, muscular soreness
Neroli	depression, sleeping problems
Orange	nervousness, sleeping problems, stress
Patchouli	aphrodisiac, anxiety, depression
Pine needle	colds, nervousness, stress
Rose	aphrodisiac, gynaecological problems
Rosemary	rheumatism, gout, muscular pains
St. John's wort	anxiety, depression, hysteria
Sage	asthma, neck, voice, gums
Sandalwood	aphrodisiac, asthma, nausea
Tea tree	skin problems, fungal infections
Thyme	anxiety, bronchitis, nerves, cardiovascular system
Vetiver	nerves, immune system
Ylang-ylang	aphrodisiac, intestinal infections

Some oils, especially camphor, peppermint, thyme and camomile, can impair or even nullify the effects of homeopathic medication.

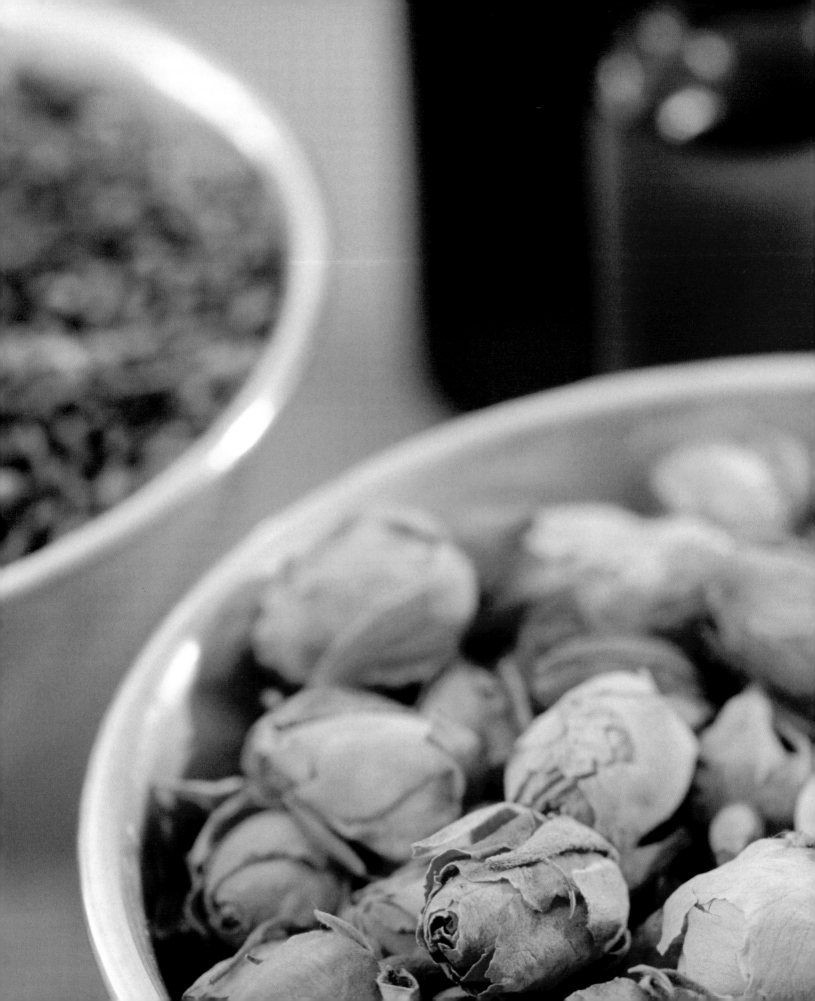

As soon as you even think about pleasant smells, your mind relaxes and your body is full of impulses that give you a sense of well-being.

Our olfactory sense is unfortunately the most underrated of the five senses. The capacity for smell plays a somewhat subordinate role for humans, as opposed to hearing and sight for example. In the course of aroma therapy, it becomes increasingly important to make conscious use of our sense of smell. In order to benefit from these wonderful experiences of fragrances for our daily health, essential oils are used. This is the name given to pleasant-smelling plant substances that do not undergo vegetable metabolism but vaporise once they are released. Almost all plants have their own individual essential oils because they not only serve to entice insects but also provide defence against bacteria, fungi and parasites. The content of essential oils in plants ranges between 0.01 and 10 per cent.

An essential oil is sometimes composed of up to a hundred individual substances that produce the unique type of scent only in this special combination. The effects are correspondingly diverse; most common of all are disinfectant, immune system-stimulating and antibiotic properties. Furthermore, some oils are specialised and have a healing effect on particular organs – for example sage, which is effective in the mouth and throat, or thyme, which relieves coughs.

Aromatherapy works by using essential oils in a targeted manner. It falls back on a repertoire of about 200 oils. These are either released into the air through fragrance lamps, inhaled, or – mixed with so-called base oils – applied to the skin. A further form of application is the bath. This involves the aromatic substances being absorbed into the body in the breathing process and through the skin. For an aroma bath, you simply add a few drops of essential oil to the full bathtub. (The precise amount depends on the intensity of the oil and the amount of water – there are small and large bathtubs!) It is also advisable to use the essential oil with a carrier substance, i.e. mix the concentrated oil with a dessertspoon of cream or honey. Some vegetable oil or neutral soap can also serve as an emulsifier; seaweed powder is also very helpful in this regard.

Just as there is no joy without sorrow, there is no essential oil without possible side-effects: all citrus oils, laurel and cinnamon can induce allergies. And if you have a tendency towards epilepsy, you must avoid the following essences: basil, camphor, cedar, cypress, fennel, garden mint, hyssop,

Perhaps surprisingly, our sense of smell is the most highly developed of all our senses. In the domes of the nasal cavities, at about eye level, our olfactory mucous tissue bears millions of highly specialised cells on each side that are renewed every 28 days. Each individual cell bears 6–8 tiny hairs with receptors into which the fragrant molecules fit precisely – a veritable wonder of nature.

sage, thuja and wormwood. Other essential oils increase your blood pressure, so you should avoid mountain savoury, oregano, thyme, rosemary, hyssop, sage and thuja if your blood pressure is high, or you should at least be very careful with the dosage. In pregnancy too you should be particularly careful with essential oils and never use the following oils under any circumstances: camphor, cinnamon, fennel, hyssop, lemon balm, lovage, mint, nutmeg, rosemary, sage and thyme.

EQUIPMENT – MAKE SURE YOU HAVE EVERYTHING AT HAND

Of course, enjoyment in the bath calls for a few implements – several soft fleecy towels for example. These can be plain white, but there are also some really lovely towels on the market with patterns that are simply a delight to the eye. You might think about allowing yourself a little luxury by purchasing beautiful towels to considerably increase the enjoyment of taking a bath. Towel warmers are a useful luxury. As a rule, they consist of a heater, which can be of various sizes, on which you hang your towels so that they will then be pleasantly warm for you when it is time to step out of the bath.

Indispensable for safety are a slip-protection bathroom mat and bath mat for the tub. Also consider fitting a sturdy handle to the wall beside the bathtub. You can slip over in the bath more easily than you would think possible – and this does not just apply to elderly, frail people. A bath thermometer is not a luxury, as you have to maintain a certain exact temperature for many baths. A bath cushion (with suckers) for the nape of the

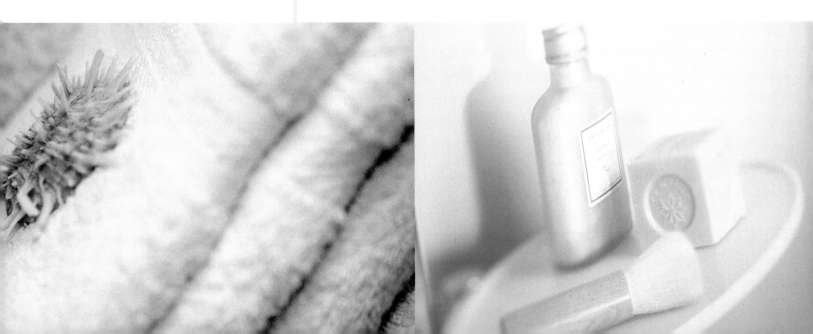

neck is not absolutely necessary, but the low expenditure is worth it for
a bit of extra comfort – and you do want to feel wonderful in the bath,
don't you? You do not need to buy a portable CD player – generally with
integrated radio and cassette recorder – exclusively for the bathroom.
Normally the CD player can also be very useful in the kitchen. For safety
reasons, you should use a battery-operated device in the bathroom.

A shower nozzle with variable pressure and a water jet is a very practical
device. If you do not yet have one, you can simply exchange the old
nozzle for a sophisticated one of this kind. A shower nozzle like this is no
mere luxury – it is indispensable for proper bath therapy.

The Shower – a Quick Alternative

These days, taking a shower has become a practical, quick alternative to
having a proper bath. It takes less time and is more hygienic. Medically
speaking, taking a shower is similar to an application of Kneipp's affusions,
although it involves practically the whole body being "treated" and not
just individual parts. The healthy effect of showering – already highly regarded by the ancient Greeks – depends on the temperature and of course
also on the water pressure. You have the following options:

● Cold showers stimulate the circulation and toughen it up. But they should
  never last longer than 20 to 30 seconds. Then rub yourself thoroughly dry.
  On hot summer days, cooling showers are very refreshing. Get into the
  shower at a temperature of 25 °C (77 °F), then lower the temperature to
  23 °C (73 °F) after one minute and to 20 °C (68 °F) after a further minute.

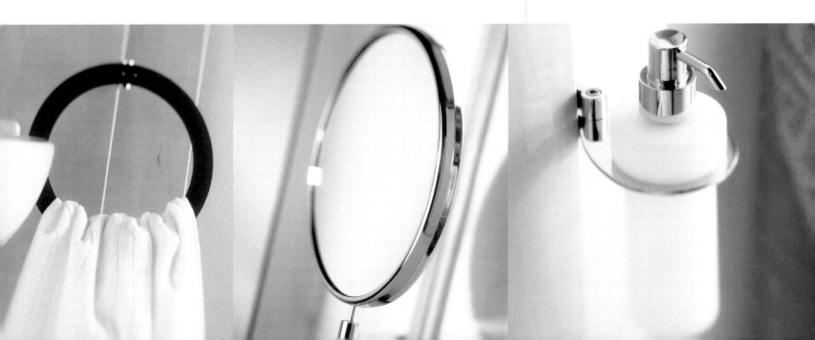

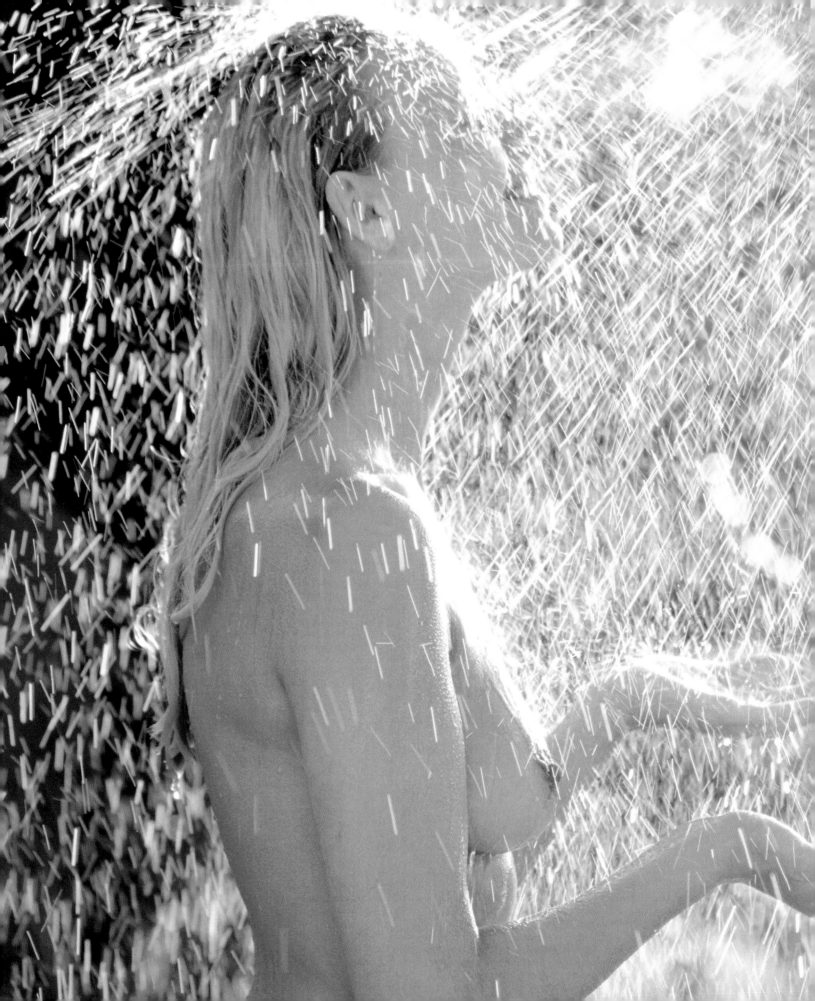

- Take hot showers at a temperature of 38–41 °C (100–105 °F); these should last about 5 to 10 minutes. They stimulate the metabolism, lower the blood pressure and relax the muscles.

- Poikilothermic showers are particularly helpful in the morning to wake you up. You should always start hot (around 38–40 °C, or 100–104 °F) and change over to cold water after about five minutes. After ten seconds under the cold shower, you should shift towards hot again – this time for three minutes. Change the temperature two to four times. Poikilothermic showers always end with a cold rinse.

The shower was originally intended as a means of allowing as many people as possible to wash in as short a time as possible. The health benefits of this cleansing method were only discovered later.

SWEATING FOR YOUR HEALTH: THE SAUNA

Complete relaxation, detoxification of the body and smooth skin – a visit to the sauna is an ideal way of achieving all these aims. Admittedly, sweating in a narrow wooden hut is not everyone's cup of tea, but the health benefits are almost second to none.

Sweating in either damp or dry heat is a tradition that dates back thousands of years. In about 450 BC, the Greek historian Herodotus described the bathing habits of the Scythians thus: "They erect three poles, which are joined at the top. Over this construction they lay a blanket of felt and draw it taut; they then cast red-hot stones from a fire into a basin on the ground, positioned in the middle of the tent. Having then fetched hemp-seed, they crawl back inside the tent and scatter it onto the glowing stones. This produces a profusion of steam such as no Hellenian bath can match; the Scythians howl with delight over this steam. They avail themselves of this procedure in place of a bath, since bathing in water is unknown to them."

The procedure of sweating in either damp or dry heat, thereby inducing the body to secrete organic waste matter, can be traced back to the stone sweat-bath from ancient times. For this purpose, stones were heated on a fireplace; the water that was sprayed onto them immediately vaporised, thus maintaining the temperature in the sweating room at a high level, which remained largely constant for quite some time after the stones had started to cool down.

The advantage of this procedure was soon appreciated. As a rule, it was carried out for no longer than 15 or 20 minutes at a time and had no detrimental effects on the body, even at quite high temperatures; the cardiovascular system was practically unaffected. The sweat bath was therefore quick to develop into something of a popular sport, which was well suited even to the elderly and infirm.

The Russian bath, the *banya*, was originally celebrated in a wooden bathing hut fitted with a series of benches successively rising to the rear. The air temperature ranges from 40 to 50 °C (104 to 122 °F). The air is moisturised by water that is constantly poured onto hot stones, and the humidity is typically of such a high level that suspended water droples form in the air; however, air temperatures of under 50 °C (122 °F) are still bearable. This extremely humid air precludes bathing in higher temperatures: the body would perspire, but as a result of the high air humidity, the sweat on the skin could no longer evaporate.

The banya gradually developed into our modern steam bath, which however is humidified at regular intervals by steam from a machine located outside the room.

In the sauna – a word from Finland, where this form of bath has been enjoyed for centuries, especially in the wooden bathing huts on the banks of rivers and lakes – the air is dry. Whilst the temperature can reach 100 °C (212 °F), the relative humidity is comparatively low; the air is only briefly moisturised by water which is poured onto the hot stones. The sauna is made of wood and, like the banya, is fitted out with benches successively rising toward the rear. One usually begins on the lowest bench, progressing to the next after a few minutes.

The walls and benches of the sauna are invariably made of wood, instead of being lined with tiles like the steam bath with its lower temperatures, because wood does not burn the skin as readily as stone. Since the air is very dry, the perspiration secreted by the body can readily evaporate. This in turn cools the skin, thus preventing it from overheating.

In the Irish bath, another form of steam bath, mist is not produced since fresh air is constantly supplied to the room. The Russian-Roman bath is basically a hot air chamber with an adjoining steam room. Between visits to these two rooms, the bather enters the hat water bath, which is also of varying temperature.

In North America, the "sweat lodge" is a popular institution; this construction consists of curved wooden poles over which blankets and skins are suspended; these are sealed on the outside with earth, grass and moss. The heat is produced by stones that are heated in the fire located in the middle of the lodge.

The Turkish hammam compises rooms filled with warm air (40°C, or 104°F) and hot air (50°C, or 122°F); the hot room includes a stone massage table. The massage is an important part of the bathing procedure.

A HIGHLY EFFECTIVE TREATMENT

But why are these "sweat boxes" so effective? They expose the body to temperature changes: it is first overheated, and then cooled down. That sounds rough, but the body in fact likes it. In the sauna, hot coals make the mercury rise to about 90°C (195°F) – no wonder the body has to get itself some "air". It does that by sweating: in this all too familiar process, the pores open and the perspiration spreads evenly over the skin. In the dry air of the sauna, the perspiration is able to evaporate well; this is essential for the cooling of the skin (its temperature rises by 10°C, or almost 20°F) and is in fact the only reason why you can stand the heat at all. In order to derive the most benefit from this sweating treatment, your skin must be clean and dry before you enter the sauna. A film of grime or moisture on the skin would block the pores, thus making perspiration difficult.

The purifying effect comes from the combination of sweating and the elevated skin temperature. Loose scales of skin swell up and are more easily released from the surface. However, this process will only function properly if you carry out an exfoliation beforehand – if possible mechanically by rubbing or by a plucking massage. This makes the skin soft. In addition, the intense heat liquefies the sebaceous matter, and in this way the blocked pores are deeply cleansed. Perspiration also causes small amounts of harmful substances to be eliminated. However, cleansing occurs to a very much greater extent via the kidneys – having a sauna encourages them to work harder.

The heat of the sauna boosts the cardiovascular system and ensures good blood circulation. The blood vessels dilate and the circulation is improved. This process improves the supply of nutrients to the body. As a result, antibodies are mobilised and germs eliminated.

When you look at the scales after taking a sauna, you will notice a considerable weight loss. But this is only temporary, because the fluid reserves have to be replenished.

Taking a sauna regularly in the winter affords protection against colds.

Ten Sauna Rules for Relaxation and Pleasure

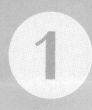

Shower First!

Water and soap are invariably the first stage of a visit to the sauna. So first soap down your entire body thoroughly under the shower and then rub yourself dry with a terry towel. That is not a mere trimming, but a prerequisite – the body would otherwise not be able to sweat at all. The usual film of grime on the surface of the skin would simply block up all the pores, and this would make sweating more difficult.

Warm Your Hands and Feet

Never enter the sauna with cold hands or feet. You can only really work up a sweat if your whole body is at the same temperature. So take a hot footbath beforehand. Leave your feet in the water until you can clearly feel that they are no longer cold.

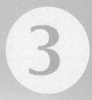

Clothes are Out

Before entering the sauna, you must undress. Being naked is obligatory here – and no one will be bothered by it. People who have never been to a sauna before and who do not understand the liberal atmosphere may be put off visiting a sauna because of the need to be naked there. But even people who are normally very shy find out straight away at their first visit that being naked here is nothing special at all. As everyone is naked, no one takes any notice.

Pay Attention to Hygiene

Take a large towel with you to the sauna. Spread it out in such a way that it covers your entire sitting or lying surface. Firstly, the wood of the bench is much too hot to sit on and the towel lowers the heat of the wood; and secondly, it would be very unhygienic if everyone were to simply sit down on the bench naked.

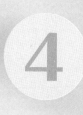

No False Ambitions

Remain in the sauna only for as long as you feel good. False ambitions are out of place here. For many people, five minutes is already enough, whereas others hold out for 20 minutes. The beneficial effect already sets in after eight minutes.

Sitting or Lying Down?

It is up to you whether you prefer to sweat sitting up or lying down. However, you should bear in mind that if you are lying down, your blood circulation can easily subside; this can cause a feeling of dizziness when you get up. To avoid such an unpleasant occurrence, you should become accustomed to always taking your time to sit up straight in the sauna. That is not a sign of poor physical fitness or of age, but a precaution to help your body adjust.

High or Low – Which Bench for Whom?

For sauna beginners, the benches in the middle are the best. The principle here is that the higher up you go, the hotter it is. So if you have some initial apprehensions, you should start at the lowest level and then advance up higher once you have "sweated yourself in".

Cooling off is Important

On leaving the sauna, you should first of all go to the fresh air room and then take a cool shower. If at all possible, you should then go out into the fresh air. The important thing to remember is that you should now take a couple of deep breaths, pumping the fresh air into your lungs. Kneipp's affusions are often provided. The icy cold pool is reserved for those who have already toughened themselves up – this is definitely not the place for experimentation!

Have a Proper Shower

To cool down, always start by showering the feet and then gradually move the water jet up your body. The reason for doing this is that the heat causes the blood in the legs to sink down towards the feet, and when the legs are given a cold shower, the blood vessels constrict and the blood rises again.

Resting and Relaxing

Each cooling and resting phase must last as long as the previous trip to the sauna. You should repeat the interplay between hot and cold three times in all. Then rest for at least half an hour.

THE RITUAL

As with the steam bath, you should not stay in the sauna for too long; it is especially important to adhere strictly to the bathing schedule with its various phases.

You should not expose yourself to overheating for any more than 8 to 15 minutes at a time. It is best to pay attention to the needs of your body and to be careful not to overdo it – so only stay in for as long as you feel comfortable.

The next step is to cool yourself down – but do this gently. Begin the cooling process in the fresh air room, since the body now needs oxygen. Then get under the cold shower and – if you can stand it – take a dip in the icy cold bath. This may sound like an ordeal to the beginner, but after subjecting your body to such extreme heat in the sauna, you will find that the ice-cold water is very pleasant. And on getting out of the bath, you will not feel chilly at all – on the contrary, the icy dip has a profoundly envigorating and refreshing effect. Some saunas also have an adjoining cold swimming pool. Cooling down by swimming is a blissful experience: your blood circulation is stimulated, and you in fact feel wonderfully warm.

The water rinses away everything that you have sweated out of your body and your mind in the sauna. The cold causes the blood vessels to narrow once more. And this alternation between high and low temperatures is the best possible exercise for your veins. The body can adjust better to changes in outside temperature and in this way the sauna has a toughening effect.

These contrast baths are now repeated once or twice. The time for cooling off and resting should be as long as (or preferably even somewhat longer than) the overheating period.

Then you must rest. You have to set aside a lot of time for a visit to a sauna – two to three hours. Next, you need to replenish your reserves of fluid. This means drinking a lot – and it is best if this does not involve an additional intake of calories. While partaking in the sauna procedure, you should avoid drinking. There is a good reason for this: in the process of perspriation, fluid – and with it the waste products – are transferred from the body tissue into the bloodstream. If water were immediately restored to the body, the blood-

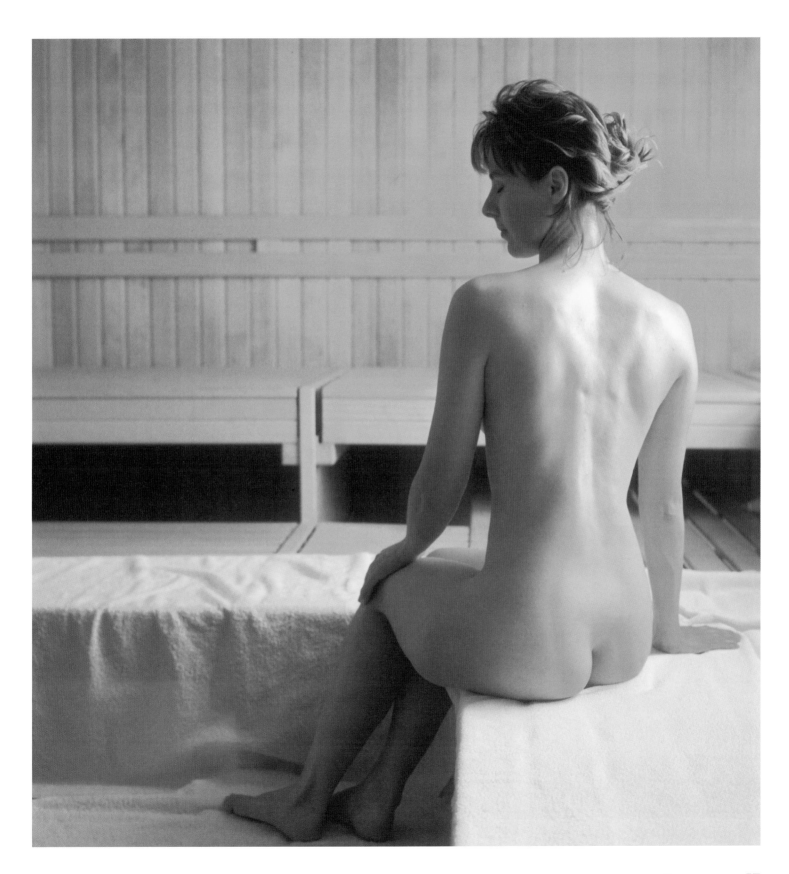

stream would draw fluid from the intestine instead of draining the tissue. This would hinder the intended purification process.

Sauna baths are suitable for (almost) everyone. In Finland, for example, even children and pregnant women take saunas. For women who are already used to taking a sauna this is not a problem; but anyone who is not used to training their blood vessels in this way should certainly not start during pregnancy. Children must get used to the temperature changes very slowly, so they should not be exposed to the full temperature on their first visit.

There is no upper age limit for taking a sauna. Even elderly people who are fit and healthy can continue to have saunas. But people who are new to the sauna should begin carefully in advanced years.

A BEAUTY CURE IN THE SAUNA

There is more to a sauna than its beneficial health effects: it has been found only quite recently that regular visits to the sauna constitute a beauty treatment. An increasing number of women now regularly visit the sauna not just to boost their sense of well-being and to strengthen their immune system – they do so especially for the sake of their outward appearance.

According to a Finnish saying, a woman looks her most beautiful during the hours after leaving the sauna. This is no mere subjective impression. The heat of the sauna stimulates the flow of blood to the skin; this in turn ensures that the skin is given a lavish supply of oxygen and nutrients. Conversely, an imbalanced or restricted subcutaneous bloodflow leads to premature wrinkling and aging of the skin. The alternation between the hot air of the sauna and the cold dips also exercises the subcutaneous blood vessels. The skin is thus better protected against unfavourable environmental influences.

Many women combine the pleasant relaxation of the sauna with the cosmetic and physiotherapeutic effects of the baths. A massage following the sauna and a visit to the hairdresser complete this all-round treatment.

A Sauna is not Always Recommended

People suffering from the following ailments should refrain from having a sauna:

- acute fever
- acute and chronic cardiovascular diseases
- inflammations, particularly of the skin, the inner organs or the blood vessels
- pulmonary tuberculosis that has not healed completely
- epileptic fits or similar attacks
- major changes to the kidneys or liver
- hypertonia
- severe neurovegetative damage
- severe circulatory disorders of the cerebrum

Of course, it is all too easy to make mistakes in the sauna and thus turn the intended beneficial effects to disadvantage. If you enter the sauna with cold feet, you risk getting a headache; you should therefore treat yourself to a warm footbath beforehand. Likewise, you should refrain from taking a sweat bath on a full stomach or if you do not have time to "switch off" after a hectic day's activities: your body must be largely free from physical and mental stress, otherwise a sauna could make you feel nauseous. Wet skin (from the shower) and wet towels are a hindrance to perspiration. Be sparing when pouring the water onto the stones; avoid doing this more than once per visit. And after leaving the sauna for the last time, do not wash yourself down with soap, otherwise you would be destroying the acidic protective layer of your skin. Do not spend too long in the sauna and do not enter it when you are overheated, in order to avoid problems with your blood circulation. And finally – wait until you have cooled down before going home, otherwise a cold will be the almost inevitable result.

Bathing is Healthy – but Why?

Water is a vital element. This substance makes up more than 60 per cent of the human body; and it surrounds each individual cell. Nutrients, enzymes, hormones and metabolic products are dissolved in the body's water and transported along with it. Water is thus closely connected with all of life's

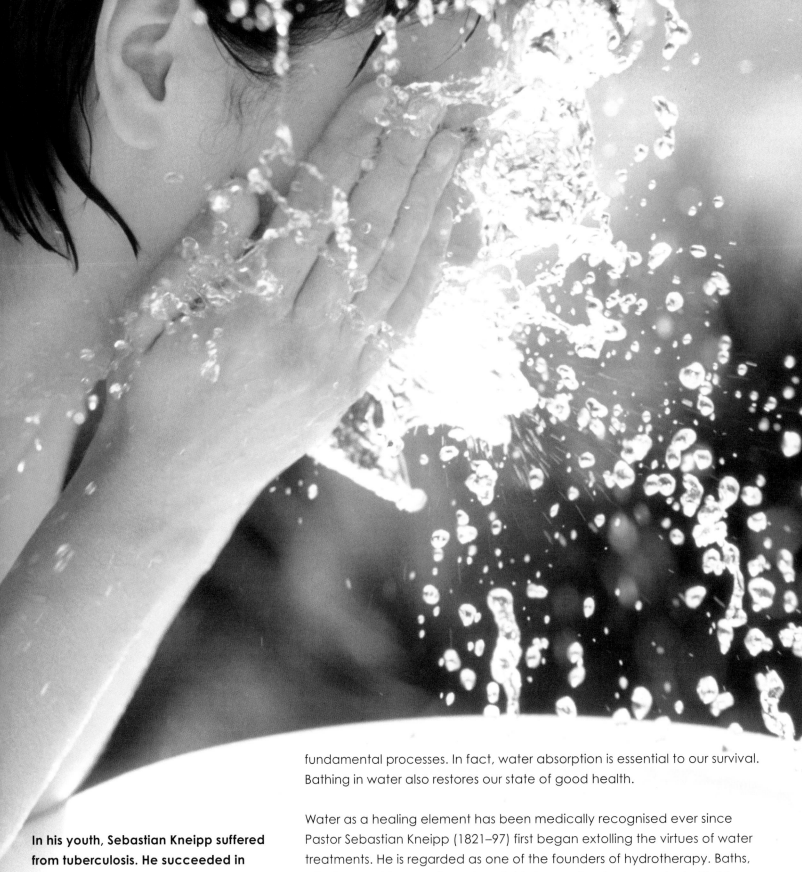

fundamental processes. In fact, water absorption is essential to our survival. Bathing in water also restores our state of good health.

Water as a healing element has been medically recognised ever since Pastor Sebastian Kneipp (1821–97) first began extolling the virtues of water treatments. He is regarded as one of the founders of hydrotherapy. Baths, affusions and lavages have invariably been closely connected with his name and remain so even today. Based on his own experience (he had

In his youth, Sebastian Kneipp suffered from tuberculosis. He succeeded in conquering this disease with the help of hydrotherapy.

suffered from tuberculosis in his youth), he discovered that water applications are a decisive trigger for stimulating the body's own defences. Essentially, the stimuli of water and of changes in temperature bring about a number of benefits:

The blood vessels immediately react to thermal stimuli. Heat causes them to dilate, whilst they contract when it is cold. So their flexibility increases if they are regularly exposed to these different stimuli. This enhances the blood circulation.

The heart and the blood pressure are also affected in various ways by thermal stimuli. The colder or hotter a bath, the more power the heart requires. For a healthy cardiovascular system, this brings about a positive training effect, whereas it would place an unnecessary burden on an already damaged system.

The nervous system has the task of passing on stimuli – such as those that have an effect on the body through hydrotherapy. These stimuli represent a kind of "training" situation for the body's own defences. The muscles relax under the influence of heat and receive stronger blood circulation – this can bring about relief from muscular tension.

And finally: through the more intense breathing, more oxygen is fed into the body – a further plus for health. There is no doubt about it – bathing is not only a cleansing ritual, but also a veritable fountain of youth for body and mind. Step into the world's smallest spa – your own bathroom.

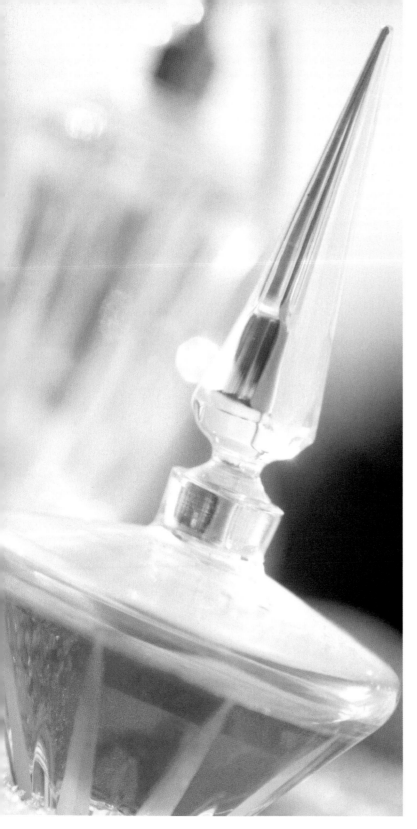

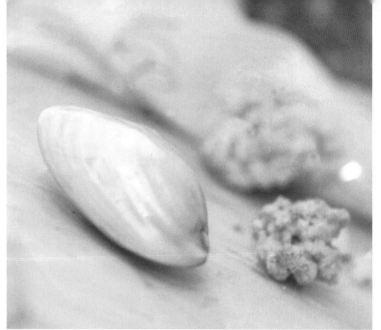

THE TIMES HAVE LONG SINCE PAST WHEN YOU SIMPLY GOT INTO A FULL BATH AND SCRUBBED YOURSELF DOWN WITH CLEAR WATER AND SOAP. ONCE BATH ADDITIVES CAME INTO FASHION, THE OBLIGATORY PINE NEEDLE BATH OR THE FRIVOLOUS FOAM BATH WERE THE ULTIMATE BATHING EXPERIENCE. HOWEVER, THIS HAS ALL CHANGED A LOT IN THE MEANTIME. TODAY WE CAN CHOOSE BETWEEN COUNTLESS RECIPES WITH THE MOST VARIED OF COMPOSITIONS AND FOR THE MOST VARIED OF PURPOSES. MANY HEALTH PROBLEMS TAKE A TURN FOR THE BETTER WITH A BATH ADDITIVE MADE FROM HIGHLY EFFECTIVE HERBS OR MEDICINAL PLANTS. ON THE OTHER HAND, TAKING A BATH IS NOT JUST THERAPY. BATHS WITH ALGAE, HERBS AND ESSENTIAL OILS ARE HEAVEN FOR THE STRESSED BODY AND MIND; THEY RELEASE MENTAL AND PHYSICAL TENSION AND EVEN AROUSE YOUR APPETITE FOR LOVE. THE WIDE SELECTION OF BATH ADDITIVES ON THE FOLLOWING PAGES ARE SURE TO LEAVE NOTHING TO BE DESIRED.

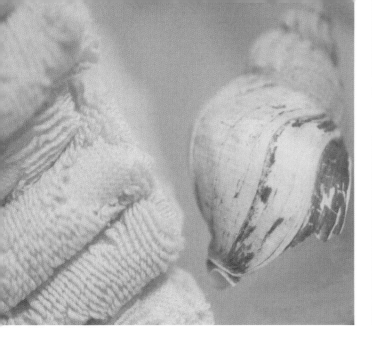

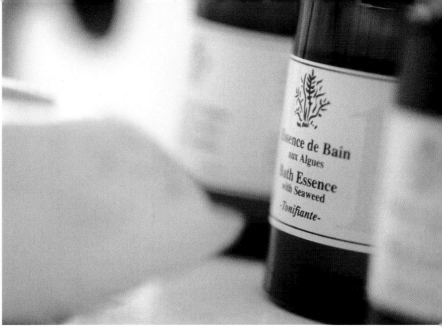

Bath Essence
with Seaweed

99 Bath Additives for Your Well-being

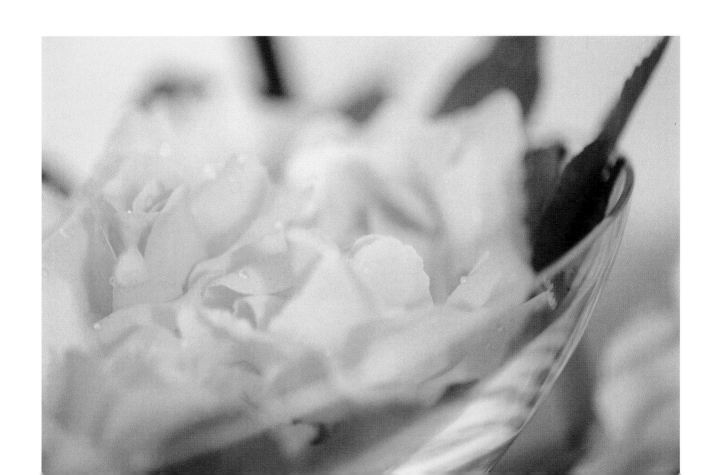

The Footbath – Relief and Therapy

You should not underestimate the effects of a footbath – that is why it is also important to observe the rules so that you can really feel good when you have a bath, rather than encouraging health problems. Particularly after a day involving a lot of walking or standing, people experience footbaths as relief, no matter what bath additives they use. You should remember, though, that even the humble footbath is a therapy as well. With the right bath additives they work fantastically to counteract all kinds of physical problems. But even with the footbath you must observe the rules.

The cold footbath promotes local circulation. It is absolutely vital that your feet be warm when you put them into the bath. Your bed for resting afterwards should be pre-warmed. And if you experience the cold as painful, you must terminate your bath immediately.

An effect similar to the that of the cold footbath can be achieved by treading water, dew-walking or snow-walking. For this purpose, you must wear suitable clothing and your legs must be bare only up to the knee. Afterwards, put on warm socks immediately and get yourself moving!

The rising temperature footbath begins at 34–35 °C (93–95 °F). Raise it by 1 °C (about 2 °F) per minute. If you have a tendency towards angiospasm, the temperature must not exceed 38 °C (100 °F); you should then also increase it more slowly. The bath should take between ten and fifteen minutes or longer, if your therapist allows. You should wrap yourself up warmly; but if you get into a sweat, terminate the bath at once!

The contrast footbath provides optimal exercise for your blood vessels if you have cardiovascular problems, neural heart disorders or vascular headaches. This type of bath can certainly have an advantageous effect on the muscles by dilating the blood vessels, but you have to move to strengthen the muscles of your legs – so be sure to do your exercises! After four to eight minutes at 36–39 °C (97–102 °F), the feet and lower legs become warm; then you change over to cold water for ten to fifteen seconds at 20 °C (68 °F), moving your feet and lower legs hard. Normally you should change over three times. Always begin with warm water and end with cold. Use a thermometer to measure the temperature; if possible, it should remain constant. After the contrast bath, go to bed or take some exercise.

Cold footbath:
5–10 seconds at 15–18 °C (59–64 °F)
Warm footbath:
10–20 minutes at 36–38 °C (97–100 °F)
Rising temperature footbath:
5 minutes at 34–40 °C (93–104 °F)
Contrast footbath:
10 minutes at 36 °C (97 °F),
then 10 seconds at 20 °C (68 °F).

The Full Bath and Sitz Bath

The full bath plays the most important role in bath therapy. Its varieties range from the cold plunge bath to the full increasing temperature bath, the hot bath and the bath that raises the temperature of the whole body. People make very specific use of these treatments for the most varied of illnesses and disorders. The rules for having a bathing paradise in your very own home are of course somewhat more simple than those that apply to balneotherapy.

The temperature of the hot full bath should always be between 34 and 37 °C (93 and 99 °F) – be sure to measure the temperature with the bath thermometer. On the other hand, people who like it colder or hotter do not have to choose such extreme temperatures; in fact, there are hardy people who thoroughly enjoy an overheated bath. But not everyone can tolerate this, and some people can develop problems with their cardio-vascular system. So pay attention to the wishes of your body and do not expect more of it than it can comfortably cope with. After all, the relax-aing bath at home should make you feel wonderful and should not become an ordeal.

You can of course also just have a sitz bath: this means that you only fill the tub to the point where you are just sitting in the water. There are also special sitz bathtubs available, but normally you would not have one of these at home.

Bath Additives for Home Use

You can gather and prepare your own herbs for your bath addi-tives. Get some information from relevant books about the loca-tion of the plants, the time they ripen and how to collect them. You will have to keep yourself well informed and know your plants well. It is not permissible to pick some wild plants that are protec-ted under conservation laws.

Only pick top quality plants that have not been gnawed at by insects. Avoid plants growing near roads, as these are sure to contain too many harmful substances. Cut the plants at their peak of ripeness; the morning, once the dew has evaporated, is always the best time. Collect flowers in

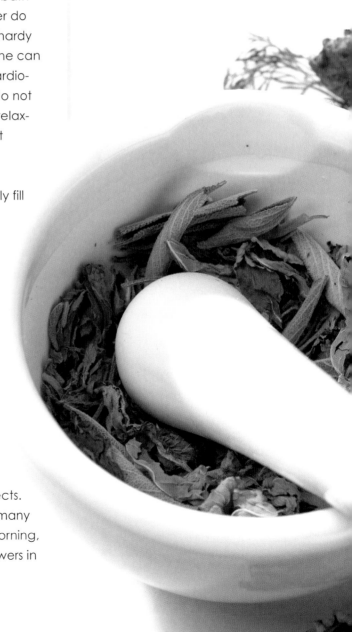

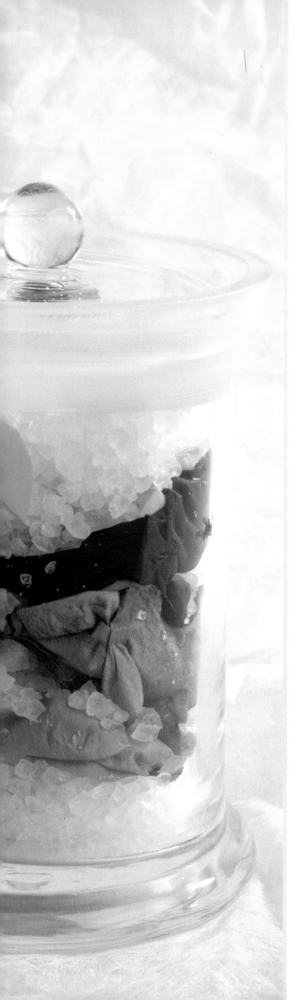

spring and summer at the beginning of flowering, the fruits shortly before they reach full ripeness, and do not gather the roots until autumn, because it is only then that they contain lavish reserves of active substances.

Freshly collected plant material must be processed quickly. Do not forget that the stems, flowers, seeds and roots of one and the same plant can have different effects!

First the plants have to be dried. If you want to expedite this process, you can dry them in the oven at low heat. Cut plants 5–8 cm (about 2–3 inches) above ground level and hang them up in small bundles in a dark place. Once the drying process is complete, put them into brown paper bags.

If you have only harvested flowers, lay them out individually on clean paper if possible and leave them to dry. Smaller flowers can dry directly in a paper bag; the same applies to seeds. Roots are cleaned with a brush that is not too hard, then dried off, cut into small pieces and dried slowly in a warm place or in the residual heat of an oven that has been switched off.

In the microwave oven too, you can virtually express-dry plants for two to four minutes. You can also deep-freeze plant juices in ice cube trays and then use the individual cubes.

How to Produce Your Bath Additives

Soak any sensitive herbs that could lose part of an active substance through the effect of heat. To do this, put them in water for twelve hours. Then squeeze them dry. Use about 25 g (1 oz) of dried herbs in 500 ml (1 pint) of water.

An infusion is the fastest method of extracting active substances from flowers and leaves. But remember – you have to use up the infusion within two days. It is best stored in a dark, cool place. Add 500 ml (1 pint) of water to 30–40 g ($1-1^1/_3$ oz) of dried herbs or 40 g ($1^1/_3$ oz) of fresh herbs and make a brew with boiling water. Cover and leave to draw for about a quarter of an hour, then pour the infusion through a sieve into a container or directly into the bath water.

In the case of berries or harder plant parts like twigs, bark or roots, you should make a decoction. (In the case of leaves and flowers this is usually unnecessary, because they release their soluble active substances more readily into the water.) Chop the herbal mixture (30 g [1 oz] of dried plant parts or 50 g [1$^2/_3$ oz] of fresh plant parts) into small pieces and add it to 750 ml (1$^1/_2$ pints) of cold water, briefly bring it to the boil and simmer until the liquid is reduced to about 500 ml (1 pint). When making a decoction, never use aluminium saucepans, as this metal could accumulate in the mixture. Use stainless steel or enamel saucepans.

If alcohol is used for a tincture, active ingredients are released more readily from the plant than with an infusion or decoction. People who cannot tolerate alcohol can use vinegar made from fruit juices instead.

Put 150–200 g (5–7 oz) of ground, dried herbs or 300 g (10 oz) of fresh herbs chopped into small pieces in a screw-top jar with a rather large opening. Cover the ingredients with gin or vodka (under no circumstances may isopropyl alcohol or white spirit be used!), seal the jar well and give it a really good shake twice a day. The mixture should be stored in a warm place for two weeks. Then pour it through a fine sieve into a dark sterilized bottle. A tincture will keep for one to two years if you make sure to store it well sealed.

Using Essential Oils

With the exception of lavender oil, essential oils are not soluble in bath water. They first have to be mixed in a solvent. For this purpose, high-quality algae powder is the most suitable because of the outstanding double effect of its active ingredients. But other solvents can also be used – perhaps green or white algae nebulisate, lyophilized seawater powder or even household products that are more readily available – fresh egg yolk, milk powder, shampoo or a neutral, high-quality liquid soap (shower gel). As a solvent you can also use vegetable oil or essential oil that has already been diluted.

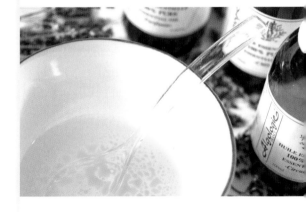

It is best to mix the essential oils – in the number of drops shown in the recipes – with the solvent in a cup or small bowl. The amount of essential oil indicated is intended for a bathtub of average size. If you have a smaller tub, reduce the number of drops accordingly, and if you have a large tub, add another one to two drops. Hold the prepared mixture under the jet of water running into the bath. In this way, the substance is evenly mixed into the bath water.

Harmless Baths?

A footbath requires very little preparation and you can have one just about anywhere you like. Place a basin in your favourite place and sit back and relax in a comfortable armchair. In summer it can be really wonderful to have a footbath in the garden or on the balcony. But be careful: certainly, a footbath is easy to prepare, but remember that its effects can be all the more powerful. This means that you must not use footbaths arbitrarily – rather, you must strictly adhere to the rules. And especially if a footbath is to be used as therapy, you must definitely get the advice of a therapist. To clear up a popular misconception: a footbath always covers at least half the calf and certainly does not reach just to the ankle.

FOOTBATHS

Footbath for Painful Feet

6 drops peppermint oil
Aloe vera oil for the foot massage

Add six drops of peppermint oil to the footbath water. Then bathe your feet until the water becomes cool. Massage your feet afterwards with aloe vera oil.

Relaxing Footbath

2 tablespoons sea salt
2 drops vetiver oil
2 drops peppermint oil
1 teaspoon honey of blossoms

Dissolve two tablespoons of sea salt in a bowl of warm water. Mix two drops of vetiver oil and two drops of peppermint oil with a teaspoon of honey of blossoms and add this mixture to the water. Then enjoy the fragrance that rises.

Footbath for a Good Sleep

2 tablespoons sea salt
3 drops lavender oil

If you have trouble falling asleep, try this footbath. Pour two tablespoons of salt into your foot basin. Add another three drops of lavender and fill up with hot water.

Footbath for Sweaty Feet

If you have a bit of time on your hands, this bath is just the thing for sweaty feet. Add sage leaves to your footbath and pour boiling water over them. Then add three drops of lavender oil. Wait until the water cools down enough for you to put your feet in it. Sage has a disinfectant effect and helps prevent excessive production of sweat.

**2 cups fresh
or 1 cup dried sage leaves
1 tablespoon sea salt
3 drops lavender oil**

Footbath for People Who Have to Stand a Lot

If you have been standing on hard floors in smart shoes all day long, this footbath will no doubt do you good. Pour 2 litres (4 pints) of boiling water over dried juniper berries and add dried or fresh peppermint leaves. Wait until the water reaches a pleasant temperature. Add another two drops of rosemary oil to the water and then put your feet in. Rosemary has a stimulating effect, and also helps against sweaty feet and promotes the blood circulation.

**1 cup dried
juniper berries
1 cup dried peppermint leaves
2 drops rosemary oil**

Footbaths for Moist Feet

Add vegetable oil mixed with lemon oil to the warm footbath. Play with your toes from time to time. If you like, you can massage your feet with French brandy after drying them – but of course, it is more pleasant if you can find a loved one to spoil you with this foot massage. This provides the feet with excellent blood circulation and they feel warm.

**1 tablespoon vegetable oil
8 drops lemon oil
French brandy**

Alkaline Footbath and Alkaline Salt Socks

With an alkaline footbath lasting 30 to 45 minutes, you can purify the body effectively. Add a tablespoon of alkaline bath salts to the water. If you do not have time for a footbath, you can make do with alkaline salt socks. Mix the salt in 250 ml ($^1/_2$ pint) of water at body temperature, soak generously sized thick woollen bed socks in this mixture, and wring them out. Before putting them on and going to bed, cover the foot end of your sheets with plastic film. Also put on dry cotton socks over the damp socks. If your feet generally tend to be cold, a hot water bottle will help. Used overnight, this therapy will purify you and neutralize the acids.

1 tablespoon alkaline bath salt

**Woollen bed socks and cotton socks
for the alkaline salt socks**

The Steam Bath

After a steam bath, your facial skin is wonderfully smooth, soft and rosy, skin impurities are hardly visible any more and you feel very relaxed. A steam bath is ideal if you do not have enough time for a full bath or if you want to spoil yourself in between times. It can really work wonders with colds too. If you are suffering from asthma or a skin disorder, you should, though, use essential oils very sparingly. Before the bath, be sure to treat your skin with a cleansing gel and then free the pores of all residue by using an after-cleansing lotion, if possible with a slight rubbing exfoliation. In this way the steam bath can be really effective!

Steam Baths

Basic Recipe

Large bowl of hot water
1 large terry towel
1 small terry towel
for drying
A light blanket (optional)
Handkerchiefs
Various essential oils

Fill a bowl with hot water, place it on the table and add one or two drops of an essential oil. To ensure that the steam can have an intensive effect on your facial skin, spread a large towel over your head – it should reach as far as the table. If you want it to be really warm, you can put a blanket over it as well. You will feel your pores opening and all the impurities coming out. Leave your neck and upper chest free. As long as the steam is still very hot, you should not bend too far over the receptacle, especially if you have dry skin. The facial steam bath should last 3 to 10 minutes. Then dab your face and neckline dry with a fresh towel.

Cleansing Facial Steam Bath

2 drops lavender oil
1 drop lemon oil

Drip the essential oils into the hot water and inhale their fragrance. After ten minutes, you can treat your facial skin with an after-cleansing lotion and then tone with a lavender lotion.

Steam Bath for Normal Skin

Add two drops of lavender or mandarin oil to the hot water. Enjoy the summery aroma and dream about your next holiday. In this way you can relax really well. After drying, a light facial cream will soak in quickly.

2 drops lavender oil
2 drops mandarin oil

Steam Baths for Oily Skin

A steam bath is real relief for this type of skin. The deep cleansing of the pores will leave your skin fine and smooth. Lemon and eucalyptus oil have a fresh touch and an astringent, deodorizing and antiseptic effect. But you can also boil up dried chamomile flowers and enjoy using them in a ten-minute steam bath. Chamomile removes oil and has a healing effect.

3 drops lemon oil
3 drops eucalyptus oil
2 cups dried chamomile flowers, alternatively:
2 drops each of lavender oil, sage oil and sassafras oil

Steam Bath for Dry Skin

If you have dry skin, you should not expose it to steam for too long; three to five minutes is well and truly long enough. Do not bend too far over the bowl at first, or it will be too hot for you. Before taking this bath, you can cover the sensitive skin under your eyes with an oily cream. Rose oil is particularly suitable for dry skin. Dry carefully afterwards and use a moisturising facial cream.

3 drops rose oil

Steam Bath for the Onset of Flu

Add one to two drops of lavender and tea tree oil to a pot of boiling water. Inhale deeply.

2 drops lavender oil
2 drops tea tree oil

Steam Bath for Laryngitis

Add three drops of sandalwood oil and one drop of muscatel sage to boiling water. Then inhale three times a day for five to ten minutes with a sauna cloth over your head.

3 drops sandalwood oil
1 drop muscatel sage oil

Correct Cooling in the Bathtub

If you find that a really hot full bath makes you sweat and gives you palpitations, the following recipes will be just what you need. Be content with a maximum water temperature of 35 °C (95 °F) and you will get out of the bath feeling refreshed.

REFRESHING BATHS

Refreshing Bath for Tired Legs

Lithathamnion or milk powder
5 drops sage oil
3 drops cypress oil
3 drops lavender oil

Dissolve five drops of sage oil, three drops of cypress oil and three drops of lavender oil in a solvent (lithathamnion or milk powder) and add it to the bath. Bathe for only five minutes. If you can tolerate this bath, you can increase your time to twelve minutes.

Good Morning Bath

1 cup dried rosemary
$^1/_2$ cup dried peppermint leaves
2 drops lemon oil

This herbal bath has a refreshing effect and makes you fit for the day. Put the herbs in a saucepan, pour water over them and bring to the boil. Wait another quarter of an hour and strain the infusion. Put the mixture in the water. Rosemary is active in promoting blood circulation, peppermint has a stimulating effect and lemon oil lifts your spirits.

Bath for Sportspeople

250 g (9 oz) oak bark
1 tablespoon jojoba oil
3 drops rosemary oil

If you sweat readily and profusely, you will really get to like this bath. Pour 250 g (9 oz) of oak bark into a saucepan and add 2 litres (4 pints) of water. Bring to the boil and then allow to simmer for another quarter of an hour. Strain the oak water and pour it into the tub filled with lukewarm water. Then add another three drops of rosemary oil that you have mixed with a tablespoon of jojoba oil beforehand. The tannic acid of the oak bark has an astringent effect.

Soft Rose Bath

Run the bath water into the tub and add one to two teaspoons of borax to it. In the meantime boil the herbs in a saucepan and then leave them to draw for a quarter of an hour. Strain the liquid into the tub through a sieve. Borax makes the bath water soft; you can buy it from the chemist. You can use rose petals either fresh or dried; the same applies to rosemary and lavender flowers.

1–2 teaspoons borax
1 cup rosemary
$^1/_2$ cup lavender
$^1/_2$ cup rose petals

Pine Needle Bath

Mix ten drops of pine needle oil with a tablespoon of wheat germ oil and add this mixture to the water once you have brought it to a pleasant temperature. This bath refreshes the skin, leaving you with a feeling of well-being and contentedness.

10 drops pine needle oil
1 tablespoon wheat germ oil

Mint-fresh Bath

30 ml (1 oz) neutral shower gel
2 drops peppermint oil
2 drops rosemary oil
3 drops lemon oil

Mix the essential oils (peppermint, rosemary and lemon) in 30 ml (1 oz) neutral shower gel and hold the mixture under the stream of water just before it finishes running into the bath. This bath has an antiseptic and anti-spasmodic effect, relieves pain and will refresh you. If you are having a shower, you also can put the mixture onto a sponge and gently massage your body with it.

Milk Bath

6 tablespoons goat's milk powder
2 drops sandalwood oil
2 drops muscatel sage oil
2 drops lavender oil
2 drops peppermint oil

Put the milk powder under the stream of water. Add the oils to the filled tub, then give it all a good mix. This is a pleasant, refreshing morning bath for hot days that feel as if they are going to be muggy. To complement this bath in an ideal way, you can use a body lotion that you make yourself. For this lotion, put the essential oils (10 drops sandalwood, 3 drops muscatel sage, 4 drops peppermint and 3 drops lavender) into 50 ml ($1^2/_3$ oz) of neutral body lotion and give the mixture a good shake for one minute. You can also apply a little of it to the reflex zones.

Refreshing Shower Bath

30 ml (1 oz) neutral shower gel
2 drops peppermint oil
2 drops rosemary oil
3 drops lemon oil

If you just do not feel like taking a full bath – which does after all take up quite a lot of time – you can refresh yourself marvellously under the shower too. This bath has an invigorating and refreshing effect and is also anti-septic and anti-spasmodic.

To prepare for it, mix the oils in a neutral shower gel. Then take a brief shower to moisten your body. Now apply the bath mixture to a sponge, with which you slowly massage your entire body. Allow the bath additive to work in for a short time and then wash it off under the shower.

INVIGORATING BATH AT THE END OF A TIRING DAY

The fruit of paradise, the grapefruit, gives us a fragrant essential oil that is excellently suited to the fragrance lamp as well as to showers or baths. Used internally (one to two drops in a glass of water three times a day), this essential oil has a purifying effect on the liver and kidneys and promotes digestion. Applied externally, it has a relaxing effect on the muscles, counteracts depression, relieves anxiety and helps you to concentrate.

For this refreshing bath after a long, stressful day, mix four drops of pure grapefruit oil with one drop each of helichrysum and pure rose oil. It will really make your evening!

4 drops grapefruit oil
1 drop helichrysum
1 drop pure rose oil

ANTI-EXHAUSTION BATH FOR STRESSED PEOPLE

Grapefruit oil is also the key ingredient of this refreshing mixture for your bath. This bath will soon make your exhaustion and the after-effects of the day's stress literally disappear into thin air, and in the evening you will feel as if you had just got out of bed! For this superb mixture, first take 5 ml ($^{1}/_{6}$ oz) of diluted grapefruit oil and mix it with one drop of geranium oil and two drops of lemon oil. Finally add another two drops of coriander oil or alternatively one drop of ginger oil.

5 ml ($^{1}/_{6}$ oz) diluted grapefruit oil
1 drop geranium oil
2 drops lemon oil
2 drops coriander oil
or 1 drop ginger oil

BATH GEL FROM PROVENCE

Petit-grain is extracted by distilling the leaves and twigs of citrus trees, for example bitter orange, lemon and mandarin. The oils have an extremely refreshing and invigorating effect.

For the celebrated Provencal bath gel, take 30 ml (1 oz) of shower gel as a base and add to it the following quintet of essential oils: two drops of pure neroli oil, two drops of petit-grain oil, three drops of orange oil, two drops of grapefruit oil and one drop of rosemary oil.

This mixture is sufficient for two to three baths. Store the essence in a small dark bottle. For the bath, mix about a third into the tub under the stream of water.

30 ml (1 oz) neutral shower gel
2 drops pure neroli oil
2 drops petit-grain oil
3 drops orange oil
2 drops grapefruit oil
1 drop rosemary oil

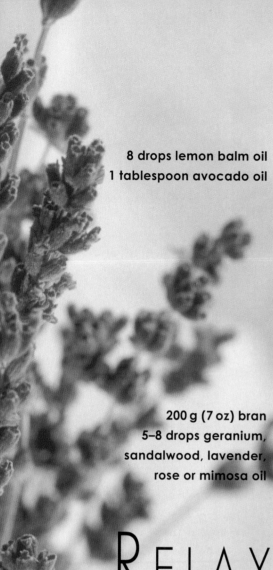

Bath for Tense Neck Muscles

8 drops lemon balm oil
1 tablespoon avocado oil

Mix eight drops of lemon balm oil with a teaspoon of avocado oil and add this to the tub filled with warm water. Take a terry towel, dip it in the tub and wring it out well. Now put this towel around your neck on your shoulders and get into the tub slowly. If it gets too cold for you, run some hot water in afterwards. Breathe in deeply several times and relax.

The Bran Bath

Biologically cultivated bran is full of goodness. In concentrated form, it contains all the components of grain that are nutritionally and physiologically important. In the bath water, it gently cleanses and makes the skin really soft.

200 g (7 oz) bran
5–8 drops geranium,
sandalwood, lavender,
rose or mimosa oil

Mix 200 g (7 oz) of bran with five to eight drops of essential oil – perhaps geranium, sandalwood, lavender, rose or mimosa – and put the mixture into a little cloth bag. While bathing, massage the skin with this soft wash mitten.

RELAXATION BATHS

Harmonious Lavender Bath

10 drops lavender oil
or 10 drops chamomile oil

Run pleasantly warm water into the tub and add ten drops of lavender or chamomile oil.

Bath for Meditation

50 g (1²/₃ oz) lithothamnion algae
4 drops cistus oil

Put 50 g (1²/₃ oz) of lithothamnion algae into the tub under the water stream. Shortly before you get into the bath, distribute four drops of cistus oil in the water. You should spend ten to fifteen minutes in this bath.

Restorative St. John's Wort Bath

Add ten drops of St. John's wort oil to the jojoba oil and mix well. Now add this mixture to the water already in the bath. If you find it cold, drink one or two cups of St. John's wort tea before getting in. The vapours will have a calming effect on your nerves and will put your mind at rest; dry off with a soft terry towel and relax. As St. John's wort oil increases the photosensitivity of the skin, you should not lie in the sun afterwards.

10 drops St. John's wort oil
1 tablespoon jojoba oil

The Home-style Relaxation Bath

Raid your spice rack. Perhaps you will find that you have a few bay leaves left over and a handful each of peppermint leaves, lavender flowers, some marjoram and thyme and even some sage tea. Use these herbs to make 2 litres (4 pints) of tea and pour it into the bath water. Inhale slowly and deeply – you will feel really good.

Laurel and peppermint leaves
A handful of lavender flowers
Some marjoram
Some thyme
A few sage leaves

Bath for Thinkers

If you think a lot and sometimes even too much, this bath is just right for you. Mix together a tablespoon of honey, eight drops of lemon balm oil, four drops of lemon oil and two drops of peppermint oil. Pour this mixture into the bath and climb in. The water temperature should be pleasant for you. Bathe for only 10 to 15 minutes at first; later you can stay in the tub for up to 20 minutes. Then relax to your favourite music.

1 tablespoon honey
8 drops lemon balm oil
4 drops lemon oil
2 drops peppermint oil
or angelica (angel root)

Intensive Relaxation Bath

Mix the neroli oil and the bitter orange oil with the marjoram oil in a neutral shower gel and add this mixture to the hot water. Consciously breathe in and relax. This bath counteracts depression, has an antispasmodic effect and strengthens you emotionally. Then spoil yourself with a vitaroma-therapie® embrocation (containing neroli, lavender, marjoram, rosewood and lemon grass oil).

20 ml (²/₃ oz) neutral shower gel
1 drop neroli oil
2 drops bitter orange oil
5 drops marjoram oil

CLEAN BODY, CLEAN MIND

The Saturday evening bath ritual is now largely a thing of the past. Nonetheless, you will often find yourself simply longing to sit in the bathtub straight away – and the internal grime is washed away with the external grime.

CLEANSING BATHS

COFFEE GROUNDS BATH

Coffee grounds
5 tablespoons fresh full cream milk
or coffee cream

If you feel that you have to relax after a coffee morning and some refreshment would do your skin good, this bath is just the right thing. Take cold coffee grounds and mix with five tablespoons of milk or coffee cream. Add this mixture to the stream of water running into the bath. You can also rub down your body with the coffee grounds and oil. Coffee grounds provide good exfoliation; mind you, the coffee should not be too finely ground.

MUD BATH

1 pack sea sediments
5 drops verbena oil

Get into the bath, have a brief hot shower and then apply a mudpack to your moist skin. Sea sediments are the most effective for this purpose: this mud from the depths of the sea is exceptionally rich in natural active substances, and as it contains crushed mussel shells, silicates and 15 percent algae (asophylum nodosum and fucus serratus) it really works deeply. Rub yourself down with a natural sponge using circular movements. Allow the mudpack to work in for about five to ten minutes and then rinse off under the shower jet. Then take another short full bath containing verbena. It is effective against insomnia, stress and coronary vasodilation.

Bath for Sweaty Gardeners

If you have been working all day in the garden, you will be ready for this bath. Mix six drops of lavender oil, two drops of lemon oil, two drops of orange oil and two drops of juniper oil in 50 g ($1^2/_3$ oz) of sea salt. Then put the mixture in the tub and run hot water into it. The higher the water temperature, the more tired you will feel afterwards. But be careful: an excessively hot bath can be hazardous for your cardiovascular system!

50 g ($1^2/_3$ oz) sea salt
6 drops lavender oil
2 drops lemon oil
2 drops orange oil
2 drops juniper oil

Cleansing Bath for Do-it-yourselfers

Pour soap flakes into the tub, run hot water into it and finally add drops of essential oils mixed with half a cup of sea salt. Straight after the bath, groom your hands and feet with a large nailbrush.

30 g (1 oz) soap flakes
$^1/_2$ cup sea salt
5 drops eucalyptus oil
4 drops lavender oil

Bath for Beautiful Skin

Put a cup of wheat bran in a flannel and allow the water to trickle through. This soaks the bran and the result is a bath that makes your skin beautiful. It also relieves itches. If you feel warm afterwards, simply stroke the water from your body very lightly and wait until you dry naturally.

$^1/_2$ cup wheat bran

Bath for Supple Skin

Run hot water into the tub – the best temperature is 37 °C (99 °F) – and mix in 500 ml (1 pint) of glycerine. A bath like this restores the skin's moisture and makes it soft and supple. You must then apply a care product – e.g. the body milk lait corporel (algologie®) – so that your skin does not have to draw its moisture from deep down. This product guarantees intensive continuous deep moisturising of the skin.

500 ml (1 pint) glycerine

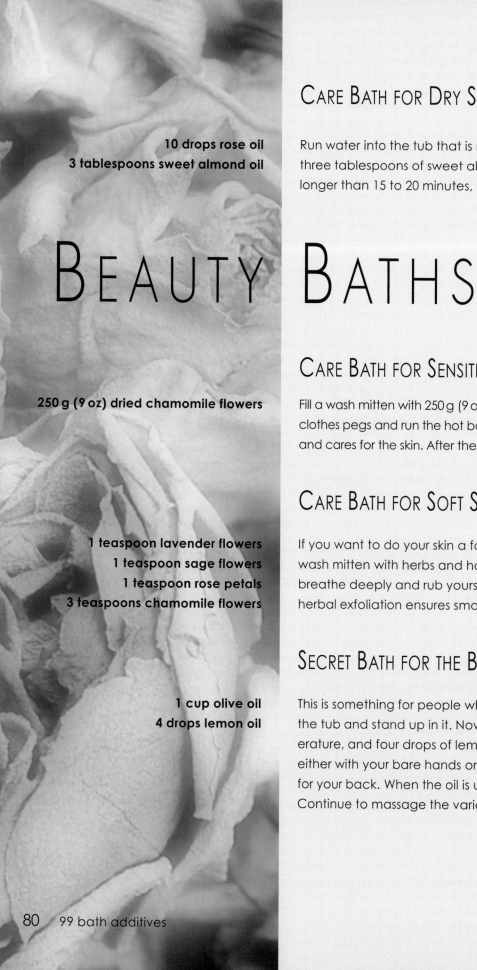

10 drops rose oil
3 tablespoons sweet almond oil

250 g (9 oz) dried chamomile flowers

1 teaspoon lavender flowers
1 teaspoon sage flowers
1 teaspoon rose petals
3 teaspoons chamomile flowers

1 cup olive oil
4 drops lemon oil

BEAUTY BATHS

CARE BATH FOR DRY SKIN

Run water into the tub that is not too hot. Add ten drops of rose oil and three tablespoons of sweet almond oil. You should not stay in the bath for longer than 15 to 20 minutes, as this would be too hard on the skin.

CARE BATH FOR SENSITIVE SKIN

Fill a wash mitten with 250 g (9 oz) of dried chamomile flowers, seal it with clothes pegs and run the hot bath water over it. A chamomile bath cleanses and cares for the skin. After the bath, your skin will feel velvety soft and smooth.

CARE BATH FOR SOFT SKIN

If you want to do your skin a favour, this bath is just the right thing. Fill the wash mitten with herbs and hang it in the water stream. Sit down in the tub, breathe deeply and rub yourself down with the filled wash mitten. This soft herbal exfoliation ensures smooth skin.

SECRET BATH FOR THE BEAUTIFUL WOMAN

This is something for people who like to experiment. Run warm water into the tub and stand up in it. Now take the olive oil, which is at room temperature, and four drops of lemon oil and spread it carefully over your skin, either with your bare hands or with a large baking brush. Get some help for your back. When the oil is used up, you can slowly sit down in the bath. Continue to massage the various parts of your body.

Oriental Beauty Bath

This bath takes somewhat longer to prepare, but it is worth the effort. First carefully boil the whole grain barley in 2 litres (4 pints) of water at a low temperature, stirring occasionally. If you want to save time, you can use a pressure cooker. Then mix the wholemeal flour and the almond meal with the whole grain barley and stir the mixture well. Put the paste on a kitchen towel; tie it up carefully and place it in the bath. Now run the water in and add two cups of fresh full cream milk and three drops of patchouli oil to the bath water. This will make your skin wonderfully smooth.

1 cup whole grain barley
$1/2$ cup wholemeal flour
$1/4$ cup almond meal
2 cups fresh full cream milk
3 drops patchouli oil

Care Bath for Stressed Skin

This bath additive cares for the skin and at the same time has a beneficial effect on your sense of well-being. Mix all the ingredients in a bowl. It is best to use a whisk for this purpose to make a smooth emulsion. Then pour the mixture into the bath water and lie in the tub for 15 minutes.

2 tablespoons sweetened cream
2 tablespoons avocado oil
6 drops geranium oil
2 drops bergamot oil
2 drops rose oil

Cream Bath for the Skin

Although too much cream is unhealthy because of the animal fat, a cream bath is bliss for irritated dry skin. Depending on the size of the bath-tub, pour one to two cartons of sweetened cream into the warm bath water together with three drops of sandalwood oil for aroma. People who have intolerance to normal cow's milk should use goat's milk powder. Then dissolve four to seven tablespoons of powder, depending on the size of the tub, in boiling water and add some aroma with three drops of rose or tea tree oil.

1–2 cartons sweetened cream
3 drops sandalwood oil,
alternatively:
4–7 tablespoons goat's milk powder
3 drops rose or tea tree oil

Buttermilk Bath

It is best to pour the buttermilk into the bath first. Then mix in the water slowly with the whisk. Only gradually increase the temperature to prevent precipitation. Do not use soap or other bath salts. Take a brief shower afterwards and rub yourself dry.

3 l (6 pints) buttermilk

Internal Purification

The sea has a highly stimulating effect on the body's metabolism. Waste products are eliminated and the body is cleansed internally. This kind of bath is tiring and you must rest afterwards. It is best to bathe in the evening and then go to bed.

PURIFYING BATHS

Bath to Prepare You for Tomorrow's Party

1 cup sea salt
8 drops lavender oil
Lavender flowers

If you have been invited to a party again and are not in the right mood at the moment, you should take this bath the evening before. It will purify you and give you new strength.

Pour a cup of sea salt into your tub and trickle in eight drops of lavender oil. Now run hot bath water into the tub. If you still have fresh or even dried lavender flowers in the house, sprinkle these on the surface of the water too. Go to bed afterwards with a good book.

Simple Purification Bath

1 cup sea salt
10 drops lemon oil

Put the salt into the bath and run hot water into it. When the bath is full, add another ten drops of lemon oil to the water. Bathe for 15 to 20 minutes at a temperature of about 35 °C (95 °F). Do not undertake anything afterwards; you will sink into bed exhausted and wake up the next morning feeling very rested. If you are too tired to dry yourself properly, simply wrap yourself in your bathrobe.

Indian Bath

Put four drops of coconut oil, six drops of geranium oil and three drops of ylang-ylang oil into a cup of sea salt. Put this mixture into the tub and run the hot water in. This bath gives you a sense of the magic of India and awakens a desire for a relaxing foot massage.

4 drops coconut oil
6 drops geranium oil
3 drops ylang-ylang oil
1 cup sea salt

Anti-cellulite Bath

Try this bath some time – it will certainly relax you. Pour 20 g ($^2/_3$ oz) of sea salt with algae (Algen-Vital® Meereskomplexbad W) into the tub and add the drops of geranium oil. Now run the water into the tub and lie down in the bath feeling really relaxed.

20 g ($^2/_3$ oz) sea salt with algae
Algen-Vital® Meereskomplexbad W
2 drops geranium oil

A Sensous Bath

Mix the grapeseed oil with the essential oils and put this mixture in the hot stream of water shortly before the tub is full. Then immerse yourself in the wonderful fragrance and simply relax for 20 minutes. Stroke yourself gently with your hands from your toes to your thighs and from your fingertips to your shoulders. Grapefruit has a purifying effect and rose oil is wonderful for the body and mind.

10 ml ($^1/_3$ oz) grapeseed oil
4 drops ylang-ylang oil
2 drops rose oil
5 drops grapefruit oil

Dual-phase Cellulite Bath

For the first phase, after a warm shower, take a cup of rough sea salt and rub down your whole body (apart from your face) with it, just as if you were doing an exfoliation. Then take another shower.

In the second phase, spoil yourself with a warm bath to which you add 300 ml (11 oz) of cider vinegar and three to five drops of juniper oil, depending on the size of the tub. If you are having this bath for the first time, you should not stay in the tub for more than ten minutes. If you repeat the bath at a later date, you can extend the time to about 15 or 20 minutes.

1 cup coarse sea salt
300 ml (11 oz) cider vinegar
3–5 drops juniper oil

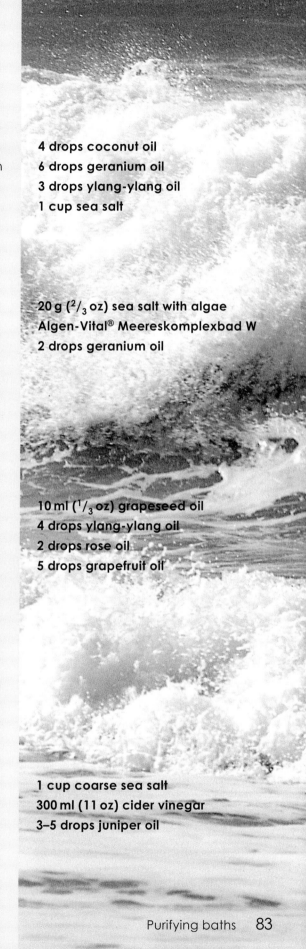

THE CALMING BATH

If you get upset easily, your blood pressure goes up and you really feel aggressive… it is high time to lie in the bathtub! The warm water and the bath additives will restore your tranquil, carefree mood. This of course applies to everyone who has a stressful life and urgently needs to relax.

CALMING BATHS

VALERIAN BATH

**6 drops valerian oil
or 1 cup valerian leaves
1 tablespoon honey**

A the end of a tiring day, a valerian bath will calm you down. It has a relaxing effect and promotes good sleep. Mix the valerian oil with a table-spoon of honey and add the mixture to the bath water. Instead of the oil you can also boil up a cup of valerian leaves and add the decoction to the tub. A cup of valerian tea will intensify the effect.

VETIVER BATH

**1 drop vetiver oil
2 drops muscatel sage oil
1 drop neroli or petit-grain oil
2 drops sandal oil
1 teaspoon neutral shower gel**

The heavy earthy aroma of vetiver oil has excellent calming properties and is effective against sleeping disorders, overwork and anxiety conditions. The plant comes from Java, Haiti and the Philippines. Mix together a drop of vetiver, the oils triad, muscatel, sage, neroli (or petit-grain) and sandal, and neutral shower gel.

TRANQUILLITY BATH

**1 cup chamomile flowers
1 cup lime flowers
1 cup lemon balm leaves
3 drops valerian oil
1 tablespoon sunflower oil**

Mix a cup each of chamomile flowers, lime flowers and lemon balm leaves. Boil up these herbs and leave to draw for ten minutes before straining the liquid into the bath water through a sieve. If you like valerian, mix three drops of valerian oil with a tablespoon of sunflower oil and add it to the bath water.

Anti-stress Bath

Prepare a bowl with green tea and leave to cool. Mix all the ingredients with the wheat germ oil and add it to the hot stream of water before the bathtub is full. This bath has an invigorating effect and also helps with nervous palpitations. Ylang-ylang is said to have an aphrodisiac effect and it also relaxes. Muscatel sage will take your mind off things. Dip cotton wool pads in the green tea and squeeze them out gently; if you apply these cooling eye compresses while bathing, you can relax even better.

Green tea
2 drops ylang-ylang oil
2 drops neroli
or petit-grain oil
2 drops muscatel sage oil
or 2 drops olibanum oil
2 drops lemon oil
1 tablespoon wheat germ oil

Calming Bath for Itchy Skin

This bath consists of two parts. First take a bath and then make yourself another affusion. Run hot water into the bathtub. Now put 50 g (1$^2/_3$ oz) of pansy herb into a saucepan and pour hot water over it. Allow this affusion to draw for 10 to 15 minutes. In the meantime, the bath water will be almost ready and you can now add four tablespoons of nori algae powder. The water should be no hotter than 38 °C (100 °F). Distribute the powder thoroughly in the bath and bathe for 15 minutes. Afterwards, pour the infusion of pansy over yourself. It will have a calming effect on your skin. Do not use any soap or perfume, and dab your skin dry gently afterwards.

50 g (1$^2/_3$ oz) pansy herb
4 tablespoons nori algae powder

Oat Bath with Rose Oil

Put the rolled oats in a muslin rectangle – 10 x 10 cm (4 x 4 inches) – and sew it up. This little bag should be lying in the bath when the water runs in. As soon as the bath is full, add the rose oil. Massage your body with the little bag in a relaxed manner while bathing. To intensify the internal effect of the bath even further, prepare yourself some rose tea. Put the rose petals, the lemon grass and the lavender flowers into a teapot. Pour boiling water over this mixture and leave to draw for about 15 minutes. A slice of fresh lemon and some honey complement the taste exquisitely. You should drink a cup of this tea three times a day either hot or cold.

4 teaspoons rolled oats
1 muslin rectangle
4 drops pure rose oil

15 g ($^1/_2$ oz) unsprayed rose petals
5 g ($^1/_6$ oz) dry
or 10 g ($^1/_3$ oz) fresh lemon grass
5 g ($^1/_6$ oz) dried lavender flowers
600 ml (1$^1/_4$ pints) boiling water
1 slice of lemon
Honey

Luxury Baths

Luxury is a somewhat problematical concept: it is synonymous with affluence, which people generally believe should be avoided at times when frugality is called for. But even if you live modestly, you should allow yourself some luxury now and then – something special to enhance your everyday life and give yourself new strength. And in this way, these "luxury baths" are the high point of life, a calculated pleasure.

A Bath for Inner Harmony

2 drops geranium oil
1 drop mandarin oil
1 drop marjoram oil
2 tablespoons almond or wheat germ oil

Mix the essential oils (geranium, mandarin and marjoram oil) with two tablespoons of either almond oil or wheat germ oil, and – before the tub is full – add this mixture to the bath under the stream of hot water. The geranium oil has an anti-inflammatory effect and is also of great help in healing injuries.

Intensive Relaxation Bath

1 drop neroli oil
2 drops bitter orange oil
5 drops garden marjoram oil

Mix the neroli and bitter orange oil with the vitaromatherapie® embrocation (consisting of neroli, lavender, marjoram, rosewood and lemon grass oil). This bath is effective against mild depression and spasms and also strengthens you emotionally.

Neroli Bath

3 drops neroli oil
2 drops lavender oil
2 tablespoons wheat germ oil

A neroli bath is ideal for people with dry skin, as it is entirely non-irritant. Neroli, which is extracted from the flowers of the bitter orange, has various properties. It has a calming effect, is a diuretic, it lowers blood sugar and it helps against stubborn coughs and skin problems of all kinds. Mix the essential oils neroli and lavender with the wheat germ oil and add this mixture to the bath shortly before it is full. Sweet dreams!

Rose Harmony

You should take a rose bath in a completely harmonious mood. Delight your eyes with a beautiful bunch of roses in your favourite colour. Simply take a rose or two, pluck off the petals and spread them on the surface of the water. A rose fragrance candle emanates a sensuous aroma. Add another five drops of rose oil to the water and enjoy the wonderful fragrance as you listen to beautiful music. If you find the fragrance of this festival of the rose too sweet, you can create a tangier atmosphere with heavy, aromatic, resinous scents.

Roman Milk Bath

Bathing in milk was already used as a beauty treatment in ancient times. Mix the full cream milk with the wheat germ oil and add this mixture to the water that has been brought to a temperature of 37 °C (99 °F). Do not use soap while bathing, because this would ruin the desired effect. Bathe for about 20 minutes and then rinse the milk off under the shower.

Tropical Flower Bath

Mix the essential oils well with a neutral salad oil and put it all under the water stream shortly before the bathtub is full. The essential oils have wonderful stress-relieving properties but you should not use too much of them, otherwise they could give you migraine. Breathe deeply and relax. You will soon notice how this bath does you good.

Romantic Rose Bath

Rose oil has been used for 5,000 years, and with its some 400 components is one of the most beneficial oils of all. It is included in 95 percent of all perfumes for women and in 40 percent of scents for men. About 30,000 roses are needed to extract just a pound of rose oil! It blends ideally with other essential oils such as jasmine, ylang-ylang, neroli, bergamot and lavender oil, as well as with tangy and resinous scents like incense or muscatel sage. For this feel-good bath par excellence, mix five drops of rose oil with two drops of bergamot oil and one drop each of lemon and coriander oil.

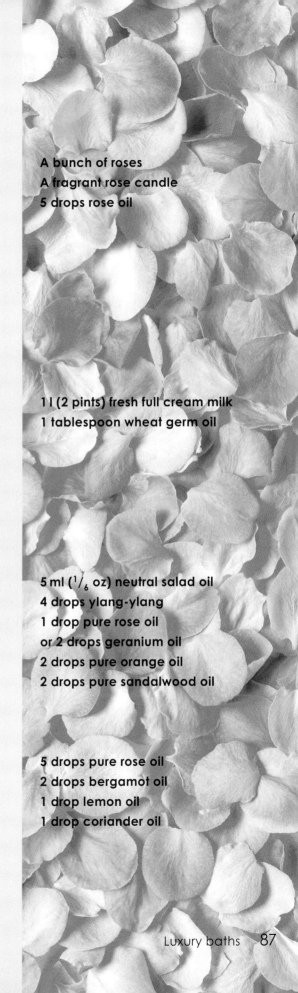

A bunch of roses
A fragrant rose candle
5 drops rose oil

1 l (2 pints) fresh full cream milk
1 tablespoon wheat germ oil

5 ml (¹/₆ oz) neutral salad oil
4 drops ylang-ylang
1 drop pure rose oil
or 2 drops geranium oil
2 drops pure orange oil
2 drops pure sandalwood oil

5 drops pure rose oil
2 drops bergamot oil
1 drop lemon oil
1 drop coriander oil

Summer Baths

A Bath Against the Effects of the Sun

At first sight you would probably think that you could do without the bath-tub in summer, because the weather entices you to open-air swimming pools and bathing resorts. But swimming is a different sort of healthy pleasure that by no means competes with the pleasures of the home bathtub. On hot days in particular, a cooling fragrant full bath is a real blessing. Or if you are sunburnt, you can quickly relieve the symptoms with a cool chamomile bath.

A Hot Summer Evening's Bath

1 cup of lavender flowers
1–2 tablespoons olive oil
1–3 drops peppermint oil
5 drops everlasting flower oil
2 tablespoons cream
or 1 l (2 pints) fresh full cream milk

If you feel like a cooling bath after a tiring hot summer's day, boil a cup of lavender flowers and strain the liquid through a sieve into the water. Mix one to three drops of peppermint oil and five drops of everlasting flower oil into olive oil or another salad oil, and add another two tablespoons of cream. If you are suffering from oily skin, simply use fresh full cream milk instead of the cream. Peppermint cools and everlasting flowers have a healing effect on sunburt skin.

Bath for Sensitive Skin

1 cup dried chamomile flowers
1 cup sweetened cream

If you cannot cope with commercially made bath salts and everything else is almost too strong for your sensitive skin, you should try this bath salt some time. Mix a cup of chamomile flowers with a cup of warm cream. Leave the chamomile to draw a while and then strain the mixture through a sieve into the bath water, once it has been brought to a pleasant temperature. Feel free to squeeze out the chamomile flowers a little. Take care not to bathe for longer than 15 minutes, and carefully dab yourself dry afterwards. If you now massage another bit of jojoba oil into the skin, it will feel really good.

CARNATION BATH

When the carnations are blooming in the garden, it is time for this bath. Mix two drops of carnation flower oil and six drops of geranium oil into a tablespoon of wheat germ oil. Now add this to the bath water and scatter some carnation flowers on top. This looks beautiful and will put you in a good mood afterwards.

1 tablespoon wheat germ oil
2 drops carnation flower oil
6 drops geranium oil
Carnation petals

AFTER-SHOPPING BATH

When you have an urgent need for refreshment after a hot day in the city, you should try this bath. Mix the soap flakes with the essential oils and pour this mixture into the tub as it is filling up with water. Do not have too hot a bath; otherwise you will not feel refreshed, but only even more exhausted. It is best to take a short cold shower afterwards so that the blood vessels can contract again. Your feet in particular will thank you for it.

1 cup soap flakes
6 drops lemon oil
2 drops sage oil
2 drops cypress oil
2 drops peppermint oil

LEMON BATH

If you only need one lemon for your cocktails, it is best to use the rest for a skin care bath. Squeeze four lemons and cut another two into thin slices. Put the lemon slices in cold water for a few hours. Pour the lemon juice into the lukewarm bath water and throw the slices in after it. If your toenails look somewhat too yellowish, you can rub them with the slices of lemon.

Juice of 4 lemons
2 whole lemons, sliced

SUMMER EXFOLIATION BATH

Mix a cup of cooking salt with six tablespoons of olive oil until a thin paste is produced. Now get into the bathtub, run lukewarm water into it and give yourself a good rub down with the paste. This gentle exfoliation removes superfluous skin follicles, makes the skin wonderfully smooth and soft, and at the same time the skin's oil content is restored by the olive oil. Once you have rubbed it into your whole body, slide into the bath and wipe everything off again with your hands.

1 cup cooking salt
6 tablespoons olive oil

Baths Against the Cold Weather

When it is cold and stormy outside, it is nice to think about a bath at home. Even in the morning in your cool bedroom, the only thing that really wakes you up is the thought of a hot bath to put some life into you. And particularly when you come home freezing cold, you are sure to be enticed by a tempting full bath or a warming shower.

Winter Baths

Sicilian Herbal Bath

1 cup lavender flowers
4 tablespoons dried orange peel
5 tablespoons peppermint leaves
5 tablespoons sage leaves
5 tablespoons thyme
5 tablespoons rosemary
1 teaspoon cloves

Mix all the herbs together. Put them into a saucepan and pour cold water over this mixture. Bring to the boil and then allow to draw for another ten minutes. Then strain the liquid through a sieve into the hot bath water. (This quantity is enough for two to three full baths. Whatever you do not need now you can store in a screw-top jar in a dark place.) This bath will lift your spirits. Cloves and peppermint are effective against muscular tension and stress; rosemary is a stimulant; sage, thyme and lavender strengthen your immune system.

Christmas Bath

Needles of various pine trees
5 drops pine needle oil
2 tablespoons neutral salad oil

This is just the right bath for cold winter evenings. Gather small twigs from conifers like pines, firs or spruces. Pull off the needles and store them in an airtight container. (In this way you can repeat your Christmas bath several times – depending on how many needles you collect.) To prepare your bath, you must first boil up a handful of needles and then mix this liquid with pine needle oil blended into neutral salad oil. This bath has an antiseptic, toning and stimulating effect on your airways. It helps both for colds and for stress, nervousness and exhaustion.

Bath for Preventing Colds

Winter is the time of annoying colds. Treat yourself to this simple but effective bath regularly – it will make you resistant to colds. Mix two drops of pepper oil, two drops of juniper oil and four drops of lavender oil into milk powder and put this fragrant essence into the hot stream of water. After bathing – you should not stay in the bath for longer than 10 to 15 minutes – dry off quickly and lie down on your bed.

2 drops pepper oil
2 drops juniper oil
4 drops lavender oil
Milk powder as a solvent

Pine Needle Bath

Pine needle oil is beneficial for infections of the airways: it helps to release and liquefy the phlegm in the lungs. Likewise, this oil is also said to have an antiseptic effect on the bladder and kidneys. But be careful and do not use too much pine needle oil, otherwise you will run the risk of irritating the kidneys. You should also be cautious if you suffer from allergies. To three tablespoons of almond oil add five drops of pine needle oil, one drop of orange oil, one drop of cinnamon bark oil and one drop of cardamom oil.

3 tablespoons almond oil
5 drops pine needle oil
1 drop orange oil
1 drop cinnamon bark oil
1 drop cardamom oil

Asian Miracle Bath

Garlic is a universal remedy: it is not just edible, it is also a wonderful bath additive. Chop the garlic into not too small pieces and put it into the hot bath water. You can also put the garlic into a wash mitten. This bath relieves skin irritation and helps you to sleep soundly afterwards.

3–8 cloves of garlic

Fragrant Advent Bath

Pour the juice of a squeezed lemon and a squeezed orange into the bath water. If you can obtain unsprayed fruit, grate the peel and mix it with half a cup each of grated comfrey roots and chamomile flowers. Boil it all up in 1 litre (2 pints) of water and strain it through a sieve. Add another four tablespoons of honey to the water – and dream of your next summer holiday!

1 (untreated) lemon
1 (untreated) orange
$^1/_2$ cup comfrey roots
$^1/_2$ cup chamomile flowers
4 tablespoons honey

NATURE HEALS

The healing properties of water were already known to medicine in ancient times. To get specific health problems under control with the help of baths, however, you will need the advice of an experienced therapist. But you can certainly try yourself to overcome minor health disorders like headaches, colds or debilities with the help of appropriate baths. And even in the case of illnesses, correctly chosen full baths can support the healing process.

HEALTH BATHS

BATH FOR COLDS

6 drops eucalyptus oil
or 6 drops thyme oil
1 tablespoon sunflower oil

If you can feel the onset of a cold or if your cold is already abating, a eucalyptus or thyme bath will help you breathe more freely. Eucalyptus oil improves the circulation and loosens the tense muscles in the chest. Thyme relaxes the bronchial tubes and helps you bring up phlegm. Mix the essential oil with the base oil and add it to the hot bath water.

2 teaspoons vaseline
4 drops rose oil

If you have hay fever or an inflammation of the nose, you can mix a balsam in a sterile cream pot (from the chemist): mix four drops of rose oil with two teaspoons of vaseline. Put a small amount of it into the nostril with a cotton bud as required.

BATH FOR LOW BLOOD PRESSURE

5 drops rosemary oil
5 drops pine needle oil
2 tablespoons avocado oil

Mix the essential oils of rosemary and pine needles with the avocado oil and put this mixture into the lukewarm water running into the bath. Massage your legs with a loofah sponge in the direction of the heart. It is best to have a quick cold shower after this bath and to then rub yourself down thoroughly with a rough terry towel. This will certainly stimulate your cardio-vascular system.

REGENERATION BATH FOR YOUR CONNECTIVE TISSUE

Put 200 g (7 oz) of horsetail directly into the tub. Bathe at a temperature you find pleasant, but for no longer than 20 minutes. Horsetail helps if you have open skin sections that are hard to heal, ulcers or burns and regenerates the connective tissue.

CALMING BATH FOR ITCHY SKIN

Briefly boil up a cup of lavender flowers and put the liquid into the full tub, then add the jojoba oil. Both lavender and jojoba have a calming and beneficial effect on the skin. Do not bathe for too long or your skin could become puffy.

HAYSEED BATH

Hayseed baths have been used since time immemorial to treat rheumatism and gout. A bath like this has a pain-relieving effect and it smoothens out flabby skin. Put the hayseed into the water running into the bath and leave it in the water. If it bothers you in the bath, simply boil the hayseed briefly, leave the decoction to draw for a quarter of an hour and then strain the liquid through a sieve into the bath. People with allergies should be careful with this bath and test out their tolerance for it first.

ANTI-RHEUMATISM BATH

Use 180 g (6 oz) of ground ivy and 2 litres (4 pints) of water to prepare a tea and add it to the bath water. To complement the bath, drink two cups of ground ivy tea every day. This herb has an astringent and healing effect. It stimulates the metabolism and helps if you have kidney stones.

To the bath water add a mixture of goat's milk or calcium algae powder (lithothamnion calcareum) and the essential oils lavender, sage and marjoram. Bathe for only five minutes at first, and then carefully increase the duration by one minute at a time until you reach a maximum of a quarter of an hour.

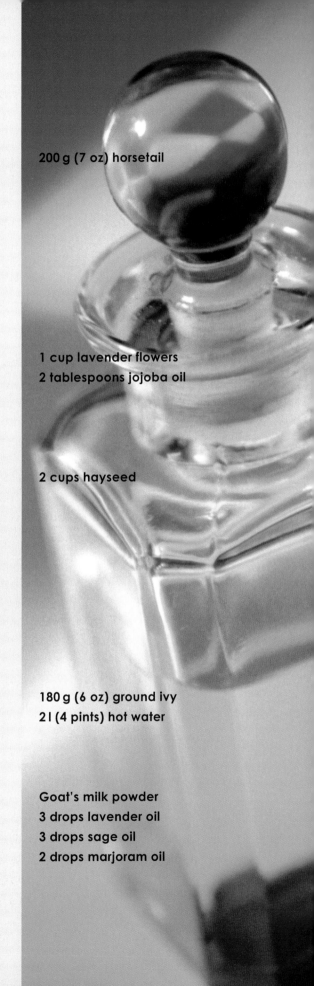

200 g (7 oz) horsetail

1 cup lavender flowers
2 tablespoons jojoba oil

2 cups hayseed

180 g (6 oz) ground ivy
2 l (4 pints) hot water

Goat's milk powder
3 drops lavender oil
3 drops sage oil
2 drops marjoram oil

The Power of the Sea in Your Own Home

The baths that are of the greatest value are those with sea algae. You can have them with fresh seaweed or in the form of powder or liquid extracts. Algae provide the full range of mineral substances, amino acids and vitamins that are gradually lost in the aging process. Without the danger of overdosing, they neutralize the acids and toxins through feel-good baths, drinks or capsules. After one to two treatments of 28 days each, purification will be achieved and you will have an energy boost and find renewed happiness in life.

Thalasso Baths

Skin Care Bath

10 drops tea tree oil
2 tablespoons wheat germ oil
1 teaspoon of each algae powder
(Macroceptin)

If you suffer from skin impurities, this bath can help you. First mix ten drops of essential tea tree oil with two tablespoons of wheat germ oil as a base and add another teaspoon of seaweed powder – it is best to use macrocystis pyrifera alga or nori alga. Mix the ingredients well and put the mixture into the hot bath water. The water temperature should be no higher than 38 °C (100 °F).

Strengthening the Bones

100 g (3$^1/_2$ oz)
lithothamnion algae powder

Lithothamnion alga contains a lot of calcium, silicon, magnesium, copper, zinc and other important minerals. In tropical seas it forms the coral reefs.

Run the water into the bath and add about 100 g (3$^1/_2$ oz) of lithothamnion algae powder, depending on the size of the bath. The water should be no hotter than body temperature. This bath can be extended to up to 30 minutes in duration – stay in for as long as you are enjoying it!

Algae Bath for Smooth Skin

To prepare for this magnificent full bath, you should have a long shower and clean the surface of your skin thoroughly so that the power of the sea can also really penetrate through the pores into your body. For this purpose, it is best to use a massage brush that stimulates the skin and makes it ready to absorb the bath additive.

The quality algae bath salt Vital Meereskomplex W is highly recommended for this bath. It consists of guérande sea salt, a well-harmonized ensemble of various marine algae and the essential oils juniper and lavender. Take a tablespoon of it for a full bath at body temperature. Do without soap when bathing. You should allow yourself at least 30 minutes' rest afterwards.

**1–2 tablespoons
Vital Meereskomplex W
depending on the size of the bathtub
and individual wishes**

Calming Sitz Bath

Put five drops of bergamot oil in 1 g ($^1/_{30}$ oz) of sea salt into a small bowl and fill it with 1 litre (2 pints) of lukewarm mineral water. Dip in a muslin compress and apply it between the legs.

**5 drops bergamot oil
1 g ($^1/_{30}$ oz) sea salt
1 l (2 pints) lukewarm mineral water**

Aroma Bath Energy

Here sea algae and essential oils work congenially together to revitalize you in general. For a full bath, pour about a capful of aroma oil bath energy into the water as it runs into the bathtub. This bath contains substances such as algae extract, rosemary oil, pine oil and eucalyptus oil. The effect is quite astounding: the cell metabolism is stimulated and the whole body invigorated. Used regularly, this bath gives you renewed energy especially after a severe illness or periods of physical or mental stress.

**Ready-made aroma oil bath
energy mixture**

Bath of Fresh Algae

Thalasso plus® spa bath with 91 % fresh algae

If you have excruciating back pains, which are often the result of excessive stimulation due to overtaxing of the nervous system or the mind, or which can also be due to posture damage and lack of movement, this bath mixture from the sea will help you. If you regularly use sea algae baths two to three times a week with fresh algae – intracellularly extracted cyto-filtraten® – you can achieve quite astounding results. After bathing, treat yourself to a pack with sea mud, sea silt or sea sediments mixed with dried algae powder or algae cell sap. This intensifies the effect.

Salt Flower Bath

500 g (a good pound) sea salt
Petals of lavender, rose, jasmine

Put 500 g (a good pound) of sea salt in a container with a wide opening, add plenty of unsprayed petals like lavender, rose and jasmine and leave this fragrant mixture to stand for about fourteen days on the windowsill. During this period the fragrant substances are soaked up in the sea salt.

For a full bath, half to a full cup of salt is sufficient. You should not bathe for longer than 15 minutes. This restriction applies to all sea salt baths, as salt has an extremely tiring effect on the body.

A Simple Salt Bath

Unbleached sea salt
Food colourings:
blue, green, yellow,
orange and red

Use unbleached sea salt which you can dye with food colourings – two to three drops of it are enough – and store in transparent jars. Feel free to put these jars on display in the bathroom, where you can easily see them: your eyes will bathe with you too!

For a normal full bath, one cup of salt is sufficient. If you have dry skin, the addition of five drops of rosewood or sandalwood oil to the bath water is recommended.

ALGAE BATH IN A SMALL LINEN BAG

Simple but elegant is this seaweed bath consisting of three types of algae in a small linen bag. You can sew these little bags yourself and fill them with ground algae, or you can obtain them filled with algae powder ready to use. When ground, the mineralising, purifying and metabolically active algae fucus vesiculosus, asco-phylum nodosum and laminaria digitata release their active substances into the bath water. You can also massage yourself during the bath with the bag, which swells in the water.

In a pot of warm water, allow the bag to swell up and then put it on your shoulders for 30 to 45 minutes. You can also make yourself a pack for your back by covering a couch with protective plastic film, placing the small bag on it and lying down. You can also pre-warm the bag with an electric heat pad under the plastic film. But don't forget to switch off the heat pad before lying down! There is no need to throw away the bags; store them, wrapped in film, in the vegetable compartment of your refrigerator: you can use them again the next day when you take a shower.

Ready-filled algae bags of thalasso plus® with ground algae Fucus versiculosus, ascophylum nodosum and laminaria digitata

SALT BATH FROM THE DEAD SEA

You can use higher doses of Dead Sea salt than of normal sea salt, as it has a completely different composition. It only contains a low proportion of sodium chloride but high concentrations of other mineral substances, for example, magnesium, bromine, sodium, potassium, chlorine and calcium. Make sure you adhere to the manufacturer's dosage instructions.

Salt from the Dead Sea

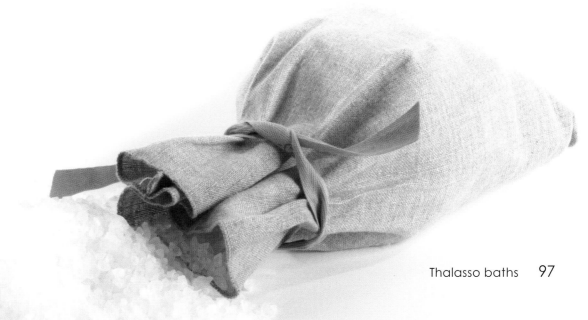

WHEN YOUR SOUL IS CRYING...

No one can be cheerful and merry all the time. Time and again, things can happen that destabilise our mental balance. Certainly, some people get over it more easily and quickly than others. Alcohol or medicines, or worse still drugs, only appear to help but in fact plunge you deeper into mental anguish. Nature's remedies are harmless and extremely effective.

THINK POSITIVE

BATH FOR MILD DEPRESSION

5 drops neroli oil
5 drops orange oil
1 tablespoon white algae powder
1 tablespoon milk powder for children

Mix the essential oils neroli and orange with white algae powder and add this mixture to the full bathtub. The water should be brought to a pleasant temperature.

This bath helps with nervous reddening of the skin and palpitations. Neroli and orange oil have the effect of lifting your spirits; you are sure to sleep well afterwards. If children are taking a bath, do without algae powder and replace it with milk powder. You should then also use only two drops of each essential oil.

HERBES DE PROVENCE BATH

1 cup of herbes de Provence

If you have a little bag full of herbs from Provence left over from your last holiday in France, you can now prepare yourself an aromatic, fragrant bath.

Put the herbs into a wash mitten and hang it under the water running into the bath. Then rub yourself down with the herbal mitten in the tub. Start with your feet, but always stroke in the direction of the heart. Finish off with a cold shower.

MEDITERRANEAN SEA BATH

Mix the diluted lavender oil with four drops of essential oil of vetiver and a drop of essential oil of lavender and put this mixture under the hot stream of water shortly before the bath finishes filling up. Lavender is not only very fragrant, it is also helpful for sunburn and sleep disorders.

2$^1/_2$ ml ($^1/_{12}$ oz) lavender oil diluted with base oil

4 drops vetiver oil
1 drop lavender oil

HARMONY BATH

This full bath is perfect for relaxation. Mix the essential oils with the almond oil, and add this mixture to the water running into the bath just before the tub is full.

Geranium oil is effective against inflammations and injuries. Its relaxing effect is useful particularly for premenstrual syndrome, anxiety and nervous tension. Incense has a soothing effect on the mind and marjoram harmonises and relaxes you mentally.

1 drop geranium oil
1 drop mandarin oil
1 drop marjoram oil
1 drop incense oil
2 tablespoons almond oil or wheat germ oil

CISTUS BATH FOR THE TROUBLED MIND

Oil of cistus is used in the food industry as an aromatic substance for confectionery, soft drinks and ice cream and as a fixative in the manufacture of perfume. Our ancestors used the essence of this shrub native to the Mediterranean Sea for the treatment of festering ulcers and badly healing wounds. Even today, the oil is still used for eczema and psoriasis, for loosening phlegm, stopping bleeding and as a natural antibiotic. If you always feel like a nervous wreck, have difficulty coming to terms with a past experience and are tense to the point of emotional frigidity, you will benefit from this essence, which warms you from the inside. In addition, together with orange oil, it detoxifies the whole body just like the lymphatic drainage provided by a gentle massage.

8 drops cistus oil
5 drops orange oil
2 drops lavender oil

Put eight drops of cistus and five drops of orange oil, and perhaps another two drops of lavender oil, into the bath water once you have brought to a pleasant temperature, and bathe in it for about quarter of an hour.

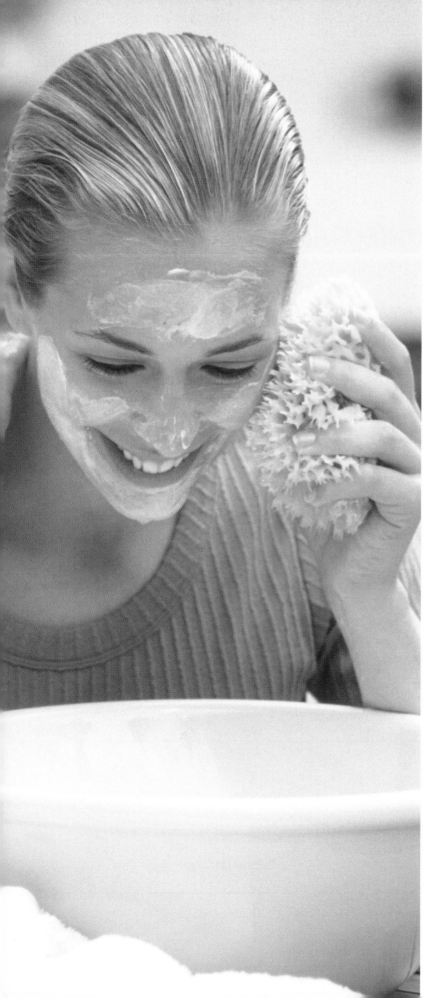
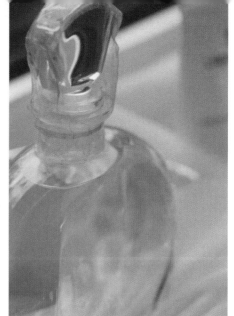
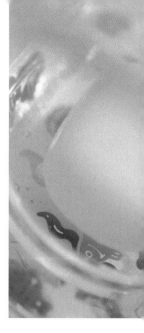

We often wish for things that simply are impossible: a body like Claudia Schiffer's, a decolletage like Marilyn Monroe's or a nose like Cleopatra's… Why are we so critical where our body is concerned? It is probably because we know it so well and therefore attach such importance to our little blemishes. The bathroom is often the scene of such self-criticism. There we have peace and quiet for a close and critical look from top to bottom, and then we think of what to do about it. Beauty, body care and relaxation are of equal importance. The pleasure of doing something good for yourself also flatters the soul. The programme for spoiling yourself in the bathroom thus not only involves your skin and hair but extends to your self-confidence and charisma.

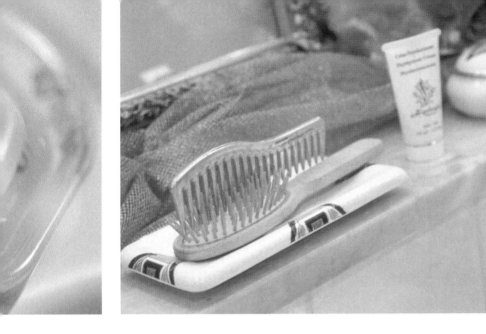
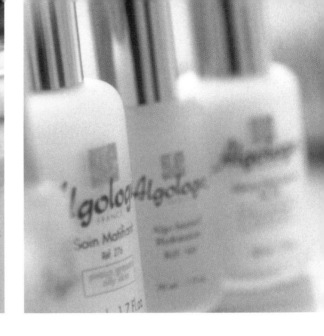

A PROGRAMME FOR SPOILING YOURSELF

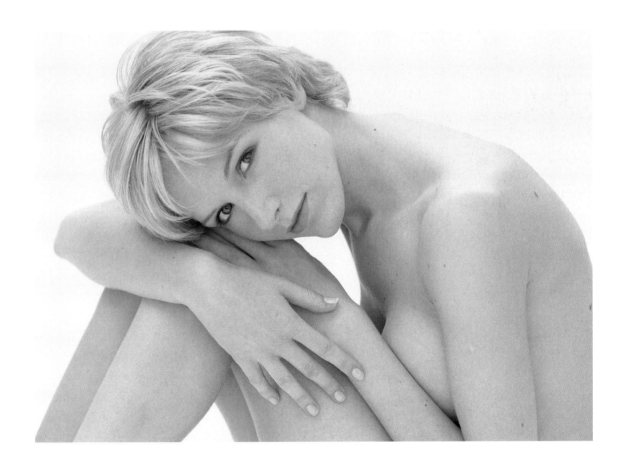

THE SKIN: MUCH MORE THAN JUST A SHELL

There are still people who just consider the skin to be a shell that serves to protect the body from the effects of the environment. But our skin is much more than just that: first of all it is the largest organ of the human body. It registers temperature. Just like an air conditioner, the skin protects us from overheating by secreting perspiration and against hypothermia by constricting the blood vessels when it is cold. The nerves which feel pain terminate at the surface of the skin, but they do not react to direct stimuli. In addition, the skin is an important storage and excretory organ; quite a number of metabolic processes take place via the skin. Metabolic waste products are not just excreted and passed via the bowels and the urinary tract but also leave the body via the numerous pores of the skin.

Our skin is made up of three layers: the epidermis, with a layer of dead cells that are replaced by the stratum germinativum; the dermis, consisting of connective tissue; and the subcutaneous layer, which is rich in fat.

The skin thus has many and varied tasks. It is a robust, but at the same time sensitive organ. So it is really no coincidence that it is sometimes referred to as the mirror of the soul. As vehemently as the skin protects the inside of our bodies from external influences, it reacts sensitively to mental stress and emotional problems. It is essentially a visible indicator of what is happening inside: the skin signals to the outside world when something is not quite right within the body. In view of the multitude of tasks we ask it to fulfil, it is necessary to protect this outer shell with special care. If it is not well supplied with blood and the pores are blocked, it cannot carry out all those important functions. To provide optimum care, however, we first of all have to know more about the condition of our skin.

We would all of course like to have perfect, smooth skin. The most important requisites for this are that it is provided with enough oil and moisture from the inside. The skin uses this to build its own protective shield, the callous layer. This outer shell covers the body like a tarpaulin and makes sure that not too much moisture is emitted.

In order to function properly, this top layer of the skin is constantly renewed. At night, when we sleep, the skin uses this phase of rest for renewal. New skin cells are created to replace the old ones. It takes approximately one month for a skin cell to reach the outer skin layer after having been created below the surface. During this time, the cells become more and more firm and stable – once they have reached the outside, they only consist of callous material.

The callous layer of the skin covers the whole body. In some places, it is wafer-thin, in other parts quite thick; calluses are to be found on the soles of the feet, for instance. Each day, about two billion of these callous cells are discarded and replaced by new ones. This is the only way of ensuring that enough moisture is present in the skin for it to be kept beautiful and healthy in the long term.

However, this ideal is very rarely achieved – there are so many things that upset the perfect interplay of our natural body processes. Apart from genetic pre-programming, external influences also have an effect on the skin's structure. Stress, the sun's rays, excessive, insufficient or inappropriate care, exhaust fumes, cigarette smoke and overheated rooms – the list of damaging influences is long. Ideal, healthy skin is a rare thing indeed. Perfect skin is characterised by fine pores, is smooth, has a rosy complexion and shimmers like silk. Its moisture content and level of sebum production are well balanced.

On the other hand, such ideal conditions are not the rule; instead we are normally faced with skin problems of major and minor proportions. These days, we no longer distinguish between the various skin types as rigidly as in the past, but we do still need some means of orientation. Above all, however, we must remain aware of the fact that our skin type changes constantly during our lifetime. And skin care should take these changes into consideration.

Have a beauty sleep – it is important not to ignore your personal sleep requirements. The real beauty sleep takes place in the first few hours after you fall asleep; this is when the skin is regenerated.

Which Type of Skin do You Have?

Essentially, we differentiate between four types of skin: dry skin, oily skin, sensitive skin – and combination skin, which is a mixture of the first three types. With the help of a simple test, you can determine which skin type you belong to.

Cleanse your face in the evening, without applying cream afterwards. The next day, press cigarette paper on various parts of your face. If a visible impression remains on the paper, your skin is very oily; but if the paper remains completely clean, your facial skin is somewhat drier. With combination skin, an impression may be made when you apply the paper to the forehead, the chin and the nose area. If your skin is normal, there are only slight impressions from the forehead and nose. For sensitive skin, no test is necessary: this skin type is easily recognisable by the red skin patches, flakes of skin and other irritations. The simplest and most reliable way of discovering what type of skin you have is of course a skin evaluation carried out by a beautician.

As we get older, our skin inevitably becomes drier – even with people who have always had oily skin.

Dry Skin Needs a Great Deal of Care

Dry skin needs care and attention. It has fine pores, is often taut and flakes frequently. It also tends to have red patches and is lacking a radiant sheen. Since dry skin is also rather thin and cannot store as much moisture, wrinkles start to appear at an early age.

Hot water, soap and synthetic soap componds also remove oil from the skin; the thighs and lower legs are affected in particular. People with dry skin should not shower more than once a day and not have a hot bath too often. It is important to replace the oil in the skin after a shower or a bath by means of oils, creams or algae centella body lotion.

Dry skin is more obvious in winter. This is usually due to the contrast between the relatively low outside temperature at this time of year and the higher air humidity and temperature indoors. Buildings are often heated to excess, air conditioning removes even more moisture from the air and rooms are not aired sufficiently. We should also not underestimate the influence of the sun's ultraviolet rays outdoors because they also reduce the level of moisture in the skin. However, if you make sure that your house or apartment is regularly aired and moderately heated, you will be doing your skin a big favour. Unfortunately, you cannot always influence the climatised air in your working environment. If you have air conditioning in your car, you should switch it off in winter.

All our body's cells need water – at least $1^1/_2$ litres (3 pints) per day, or even better 2 litres (4 pints) or more. Two hormones, vasopressine and aldosterone, regulate the water balance. Aldosterone controls the balance of sodium and potassium. Both of these minerals are essential for the proper distribution of water in the body. By regulating the osmotic pressure of the body fluids within the tissue, they also influence the tissue's elasticity and the condition of the muscles. To support the function of both these hormones it is, however, not enough just to drink adequate amounts of liquid: the water must also be retained in the body.

From the age of twenty onwards, the body loses more and more water. This moisture loss is especially noticeable in the epidermis, and is associated with a reduction in mineral salts and dermal electrolytes. These molecules are responsible for giving the skin its natural moisture.

It is not an easy matter to find the ideal product to suit your personal needs. Get professional advice before you make a wrong decision.

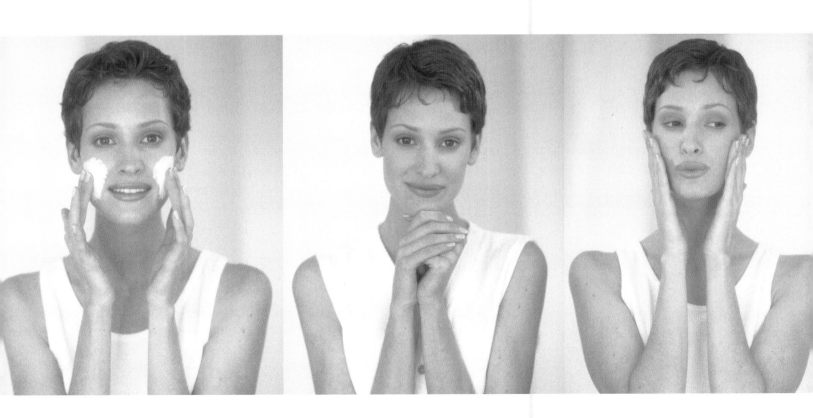

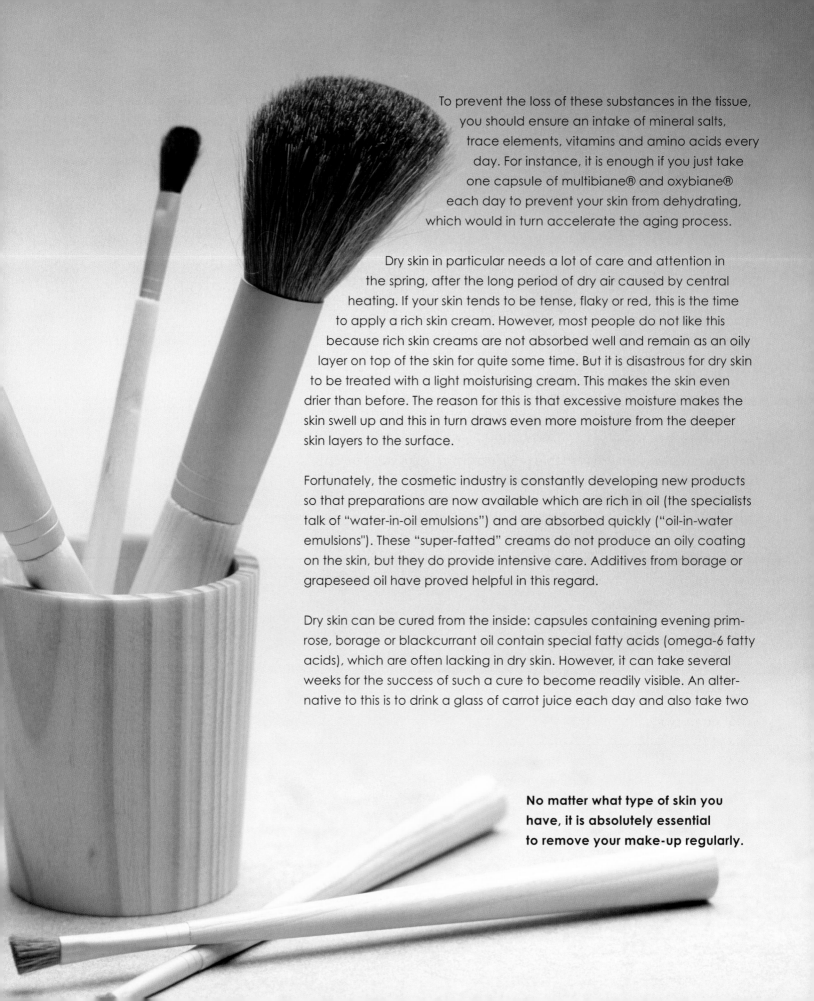

To prevent the loss of these substances in the tissue, you should ensure an intake of mineral salts, trace elements, vitamins and amino acids every day. For instance, it is enough if you just take one capsule of multibiane® and oxybiane® each day to prevent your skin from dehydrating, which would in turn accelerate the aging process.

Dry skin in particular needs a lot of care and attention in the spring, after the long period of dry air caused by central heating. If your skin tends to be tense, flaky or red, this is the time to apply a rich skin cream. However, most people do not like this because rich skin creams are not absorbed well and remain as an oily layer on top of the skin for quite some time. But it is disastrous for dry skin to be treated with a light moisturising cream. This makes the skin even drier than before. The reason for this is that excessive moisture makes the skin swell up and this in turn draws even more moisture from the deeper skin layers to the surface.

Fortunately, the cosmetic industry is constantly developing new products so that preparations are now available which are rich in oil (the specialists talk of "water-in-oil emulsions") and are absorbed quickly ("oil-in-water emulsions"). These "super-fatted" creams do not produce an oily coating on the skin, but they do provide intensive care. Additives from borage or grapeseed oil have proved helpful in this regard.

Dry skin can be cured from the inside: capsules containing evening prim-rose, borage or blackcurrant oil contain special fatty acids (omega-6 fatty acids), which are often lacking in dry skin. However, it can take several weeks for the success of such a cure to become readily visible. An alternative to this is to drink a glass of carrot juice each day and also take two

No matter what type of skin you have, it is absolutely essential to remove your make-up regularly.

capsules of wheatgerm oil. Also available are ampoule drinks that moisturise dry skin from the inside – for example with liquid algae. Add one ampoule to $1^1/_2$ litres (3 pints) of water and drink this mixture during the course of the day.

OILY SKIN IS ROBUST AND FREE FROM WRINKLES

Oily skin has large pores and tends to produce blackheads. It is shiny, because it produces a surplus of sebum; and it appears thicker, as it can store more oil and moisture. Although this does not sound very pleasant, it does have one great advantage: oily skin is more robust than dry skin and does not wrinkle as easily.

It is especially important to clean oily skin thoroughly. Although it is more resistant to the effects of the environment, it can react sensitively to the body's own sebum and sweat. So the most important thing is to clean the skin thoroughly, as this removes oil. Synthetic soaps and cleaning gels are very good for this purpose; the same applies to pads soaked with active ingredients to remove surplus oil and bacteria. Soap, on the other hand, leaves a film on the skin, especially if it is not thoroughly rinsed off; this in turn can cause pimples and blackheads. Regular peeling and showering are good for oily skin.

If your skin is inflamed, you will have to do more than just get rid of excess oil. You will have to carefully remove the callous layer and clean the pores so deep that the sebum can flow out. A deep cleansing cream is ideal for thoroughly cleaning the pores. To open the pores, submerge a face cloth in hot water, place it briefly over the skin and immediately apply a thick layer of cream, massage this in and then carefully remove the excess. Then rinse the skin with warm water and apply a cleansing lotion. After this treatment you can use normal skin care cream during the day. At night, your skin should ideally be able to breathe, but make sure to apply sufficient lotion so that its water-binding properties remain intact.

Doctors often prescribe antibiotics for bad cases of acne. Pustules and tubercles are often treated with hormones. This treatment is not without risk, as the therapy influences the brain's hormonal control centre. Before

Sometimes the cause of dry skin has nothing to do with a fat deficiency; the problem could be a lack of urea, a natural moisture binding agent. There are special creams containing this substance. According to experts, a significant improvement in the structure of the skin can be seen within just three days.

resorting to such drastic measures, you should examine the possibility of using natural products. Oxybiane capsules with zinc or zinc orotate (20–30 mg per day), pumpkin seed oil and drink ampoules with algae cytofiltrate often work wonders.

Excessive washing can damage oily skin, because it then dries out and forms more sebum to balance out the apparent loss.

However, oily skin occasionally needs cream. Although the skin produces sufficient oil itself, it is often lacking moisture. Oil-free products are best suited for the care of oily skin. There are highly effective algae products available which generally bring about an improvement in the skin within a short time.

Sensitive Skin: Never Irritate it!

Skin that very quickly becomes tense and red is especially sensitive. Its own protective system is particularly susceptible and can very easily be put out of its natural balance. The skin can then only regain this balance with a very specific regime of care. But what do we really mean by "sensitive"? Sensitive skin is characterised by fine pores and is thin and dry. It usually appears pale, with extended veins. Around 70 percent of all women maintain that they have sensitive skin. Of course, this is responsible for the boom in "mild" cosmetics. In fact, however, dry skin is sensitive and reacts unfavourably to certain ingredients.

If you have sensitive skin, you need especially thorough care to provide it with additional oil and moisture. Once it is well moisturised, it becomes soft and supple so that any germs, perfumes or bacteria that penetrate the skin cannot cause damage.

It is very important not to irritate sensitive skin. Perfumes can cause problems in this respect: if creams or bath additives are too highly perfumed, they are seldom any use to people with sensitive skin. Try the smell test: if a product smells too intensively it could irritate the skin. Preservatives can also cause irritation: after all, the substances that kill germs in care products (to make them as durable as possible) can also harm the skin. It is advisable

Are you allergic? Test your reactions. Any natural beauty product can cause allergic reactions in some people. It is therefore advisable to test home-made care products beforehand. Before applying the product to large areas of skin, test a small amount in the crook of your arm and leave it on overnight. If there is no redness or itching (or any other skin irritation) the next morning, you can use the recipe without any worry.

to obtain information on the ingredients of the various care products and the effects attributed to them. Emulsifiers based on surfactants – cleansing agents – can dry out the skin and make it rough. Make sure you know what you are buying. On the other hand, certain emulsifiers such as cephaline, lecithin and alginate are harmless. Essential oils are often used in natural cosmetics, but they often have the disadvantage of penetrating deep into the skin, where they can trigger undesired reactions. Fruit acids make the skin thinner – and thus also more sensitive. You should not use them too often.

Having sensitive skin does not necessarily mean that you have allergic reactions. On the other hand, if you are susceptible to allergies, the skin often reacts as well. Once you have found a suitable form of skin care, you should therefore stick with it and not risk any experiments.

Normal Skin: the Lucky Few

Normal skin is characterised by fine pores, is smooth and has a pink complexion; this perfect picture is not blemished by oily zones. Moisture and sebum production are harmoniously balanced. However, ideal conditions such as these are generally only to be found in young skin. With increasing age, even normal skin gradually becomes drier and thus new problems arise. You do not have to take any particular care of normal skin, but you should definitely take some steps to counteract the body's biological aging process.

Peeling Frees the Skin

Our skin renews itself about every twenty-eight days. However, the older we get, the slower this process becomes and more and more dead skin cells thus accumulate on the surface of the skin, making it appear rough and dull. This layer must be removed gently. The method used for doing this is called peeling. Regular peeling supports the skin in its natural regeneration process.

Gentle peeling products cannot work in too deeply, nor are they intended to do so.

There are several different variations of peeling, and you should choose the one that is best suited to the type of skin you have. A fundamental distinction is made between face peeling and body peeling. While ideally the whole body should be treated before a bath, it is better to treat the more sensitive skin on your face afterwards.

The simplest method of peeling is the mechanical variant. The lotion contains minute abrasive particles that are massaged into the surface of the skin in a circular motion, loosening the dead skin cells. One can use ready-made products, where the abrasive particles generally consist of wax. A simple and rapid body peeling is effected by a soap that peels the skin gently with algae particles.

Biological peeling products work on the basis of ferments and enzymes. They are highly effective and should only be used by a trained beautician.

BRUSH YOUR SKIN CLEAN

The moistened skin can also be peeled with a body brush or with a massage sponge or glove. In this case, treat your body with small circular movements, which will remove the excess scales of skin. However, if you have sensitive skin it is better to only work with a towel or a soft sponge, so as not to irritate your skin. Also recommended is so-called "Indian silk peeling", in which the skin is treated by tiny loops of silk on a massage glove.

The most thorough but at the same time most strenuous variant of body peeling is the dry brush massage, which by way of exception is performed on dry skin. In addition to removing surplus skin particles, it also stimulates the flow of lymph. Dry brushing has an effect on the body comparable to that of 20 minutes of gymnastics or a massage.

Always start the brush massage at the soles of your feet, and from there work along your legs, making your way upwards (in the direction of your heart). Massage the individual parts of your body with large sweeping motions. Once you have massaged your legs, move on to your arms and chest. Always massage towards the heart.

Finally dry brush your stomach with clockwise circular movements. The next step is to have a warm shower, and after drying yourself apply a moisturising emulsion to the skin.

THE FACE: THE BODY'S VISITING CARD

A well cared-for face is your visiting card. Like no other part of your body, your face is subject to the effects of the wind and the sun as well as car exhaust fumes and other environmental toxins. For this reason your face requires special care, cleansing and protection.

After a relaxing bath you can turn your attention to intensive beauty care. This is the right time for a face care treatment, for example. A thorough cleansing is the decisive factor, and the bath that you have just had is the perfect preparation: your skin is warm and well supplied with blood, and it is ready to absorb all the caring substances that you are about to apply. The first step is facial peeling. From the wide range of high-quality care products available, choose a peeling product to suit your skin type.

CLEANSING PASTE FOR OILY SKIN

The "combination" skin type and oily facial skin require a different sort of care. A useful aid is a cleansing paste that you can make from almond bran and milk. This is used once a week. Mix 250 ml (9 oz) of full cream milk with one cup of almond bran and 30 ml (1 oz) of almond oil. Apply this paste to your

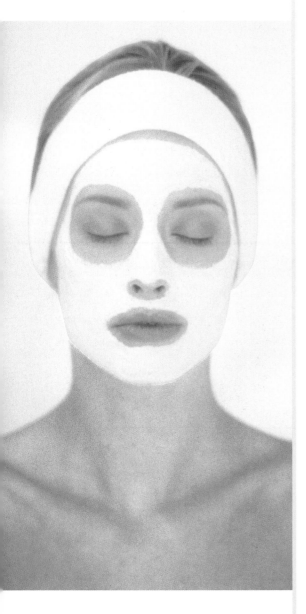

face immediately, leaving the area around your eyes free. Massage the paste into your face with small circular movements and then rinse it off with warm water. If carried out thoroughly, this treatment will remove dirt particles and cosmetic residue from the skin. At the same time, this skin care is mild and gentle.

FACIAL PEELING

Another method of cleansing is facial peeling. Depending on the type of skin you have, this can be done up to three times a week. However, as a rule of thumb – the more sensitive and drier the skin, the less frequently and more carefully this peeling treatment should be carried out.

Spread a pea-sized portion of peeling gel or cream over your moist face and massage the gel or cream into the skin with small circular movements. Pay special attention when massaging it into the areas of your face with the greatest concentration of open pores and sebaceous glands: your forehead, chin and nose.

FOR OPTIMAL SKIN CARE: CREAMS, PACKS AND MASKS

Dab your face dry with a soft towel and pamper the skin with a gentle cream or lotion. Natural substances are especially good for this purpose, as they provide the skin with moisture and nutrients. Ready-made creams can also be refined by adding nutrients. For example, mix a generous tablespoon of your nourishing cream – preferably a naturally based mixture – with an equal amount of yoghurt, milk curds, lemon juice or honey. Choose the additives to suit your skin type.

For oily skin, a mixture of nourishing cream and yoghurt is best. For dry skin, a banana variant is usually more suitable: to make this, mash a ripe banana and mix it with a teaspoon of nourishing cream. Now add a teaspoon of olive oil. Sensitive skin can be cared for with fresh frothy avocado cream: to make this, separate the yolk and the white of an egg and beat the white until it is firm. Mix the yolk with 30 ml (1 oz) of avocado oil and then add a pinch of salt and a teaspoonful each of lemon juice and cider vinegar. Carefully fold this into the beaten eggs and store in clean jars in a cool place.

How to Apply Packs and Masks

- Before beginning any mask treatment, you must clean your face thoroughly. This makes the skin more supple and ready to absorb the ingredients. It is better still if you warm your face with compresses prior to applying the mask.

- Creams and pastes are best applied with a soft spatula or a wide brush; however, never apply them to your eyes, your mouth or your neck. You should treat these sensitive zones separately: for instance, you could place moist, warm camomile tea bags on your eyes to relax them or you could cream your lips with pomade. While doing this, it is advisable to use a hair band to keep your hair out of your face.

- Always apply the mask cream to the chin first, before working your way over your cheeks and up to your forehead. Then apply it from the upper part of your nose to just below your eyes and finally to the bridge of your nose. If you intend to treat your neck, then spread the cream on the sides of your neck only.

- Leave the mask or pack on your face for around 10 to 20 minutes. Simply relax while it is being absorbed into your skin, and feel how it is doing you good.

- Afterwards, soften the mask with a natural sponge soaked in lukewarm water and then cleanse your face, also with lukewarm water. Finally, pat your face dry with a soft towel.

Facial masks and packs are an alternative to creams. These provide the skin with all the substances that it urgently requires. You can also work with quite a number of natural additives to make your own care recipes – or reach for tried and tested ready-made products.

Masks and packs are traditional beauty treatments that have an immediate effect. However, they can only of be lasting value when used regularly. As they form a film on the skin, they should never be applied when you are in the bath; so it is best to apply them either before your bath or afterwards. In former times, people went to bed with a mask, but nowadays masks are so highly active that this is no longer necessary.

Cucumber Mask

The cucumber mask is the absolute classic facemask. All you have to do is relax for 20 minutes with slices of cucumber on your face, but this vitalising and refreshing treatment is only suitable for oily skin. For combination skin you should only apply the cucumber to the areas that are dry.

EXPRESS MASK FOR COMBINATION SKIN

1 drop essential lavender oil
1 drop essential rosemary oil
15 ml ($^1/_2$ oz) pure honey

Mix one drop each of essential oils of lavender and rosemary with 15 ml ($^1/_2$ oz) of pure honey. Apply this mixture to your face in a thin layer. Of course, you should avoid applying it to your eyes. Remove the mask after 15 to 20 minutes and spray your face with *Embrun de mer* (sea spray). Allow your face to dry off by itself; do not dry it with a towel.

NOURISHING FRAGRANT MASK

4 slices banana
5 ml ($^1/_6$ oz) diluted jasmine oil

Mash four slices of ripe banana with a fork and add 5 ml ($^1/_6$ oz) of diluted jasmine oil drop by drop. Mix until it reaches a homogeneous consistency.

This facial mask nourishes and moisturises the skin, lightens your complexion and the addition of jasmine tones the skin. Remove the mask after 15 to 20 minutes with two natural sponges that you have soaked in lukewarm water.

Remember that jasmine should not be used – even as an infusion – during pregnancy or if you are breastfeeding: jasmine stimulates the uterus and can reduce milk production.

HONEY CREAM MASK

2 teaspoons honey
2 tablespoons sour cream
$^1/_2$ cup wheatgerm flakes

Sometimes the simplest things are also the best, especially if you want to treat dry or sensitive facial skin. You will often have no problem finding suitable ingredients in your refrigerator – for a honey cream mask, for example. To make this, mix two teaspoons of honey with two tablespoons of sour cream. Then add several flakes of wheatgerm to form a thick paste. Allow this to work in for a quarter of an hour and then rinse off with lukewarm water.

Avocado Moisturising Mask

You can make a moisturising mask for dry facial skin from egg and avocado: remove the flesh from half an avocado and mash it up with a fork. Now separate an egg and mix the yolk with the avocado. Blend these ingredients well and add a few drops of lemon juice. Spread the paste evenly over your face and allow to work in for about 20 minutes. Then rinse off with lukewarm water.

$^1/_2$ avocado
1 egg yolk
1 teaspoon lemon juice

Parsley Mask

Sensitive skin appreciates parsley. To make a mask, mix a bundle of freshly chopped parsley with three to four tablespoons of milk curds. Apply the paste; allow it to work in for 30 minutes and then rinse off with lukewarm water.

1 bunch parsley
3–4 tablespoons milk curd

Potato Mask

This mask is nature in its purest form: boil three new potatoes until they become soft. Add three tablespoons of brewer's yeast, two teaspoons of natural yoghurt and 5 ml ($^1/_6$ oz) of diluted juniper oil. Apply the paste and allow it to work in for 15 to 20 minutes before rinsing it off.

3 new potatoes
2 teaspoons brewer's yeast
2 teaspoons natural yoghurt
5 ml ($^1/_6$ oz) diluted juniper oil

Highly Effective: Relaxation Packs

Relaxation masks are a highly effective treatment and are usually provided by experienced beauticians. Several preparations are also available for home use.

Peloids are organic and inorganic substances that have been formed over the course of thousands of years both on land and under water. These include liquid mud and peat, healing earth, lime and clay. However, a peloid mask is only the basis, to which fruits are added according to your skin type and individual skin problems. For instance, kiwi fruits are very popular because they mineralise the tissue, while bilberries are used for their disinfecting properties. Peloid packs – as ready-made products – are mixed with warm water; the fruit is then added and the mixture applied to the face.

The anti-stress mask cools and provides deep relaxation. An alginate pack is applied on top of a basis of various essential oils, whose composition depends on the skin type.

The sea mask smells of holidays at the seaside and is practically a vacation for the skin. Extracts from mussels and oysters are stirred into a paste made from algae. This is a highly effective mask, which has an unrivalled effect on the skin. The combination is a unique mixture of natural materials as only the sea can offer.

Beauty Tips for the Face

Here you will find the most important tips for facial care – from your eyes to your teeth.

Eye Care: as Gentle as Possible!

Your eyes are one of your most attractive facial features and therefore deserve special attention. The area around the eyes is one of the most sensitive areas of the face. To prevent irritation, avoid applying creams, packs and masks to this sensitive region. Gentle care, however, is an absolute must.

Swollen upper and lower lids are often caused by weak connective tissue, so that a congestion of lymph can cause an oedema. There can be many reasons for this. Hormonal fluctuations are one possibility. The draining of lymph can also be impeded by lack of movement at night: the longer you sleep, the more pronounced the swelling can be. There is only one solution for this: do not apply rich skin creams to the eyes but only a gel, reduce the salt intake in your food and do not drink much after about 5 p.m. Lymph drainage can be promoted by putting extra pillows under your head. If the swelling does not subside at all during the day or night, too much fatty tissue is already stored in the eyelids; in this case only cosmetic surgery can help.

In such cases, an inflammation of the eyes should not be ruled out. If your eyes are not just swollen, but also red, and if there is secretion present in the corner of the eyes, you should consult your doctor or an eye specialist.

Here's how to treat puffy eyelids. After thoroughly cleaning them – there should be no cleansing milk residue on the skin – put some delymphing extract on to a thin gauze or cotton wool compress and place this over the puffy part of the eyelid for at least five minutes. Then massage the rest gently into the skin.

However, there are quite a number of relieving measures that you can undertake yourself:

Cool compresses are a relief. Fold ice cubes into a handkerchief and put this compress over your eyes. Then gently massage this area of your face in a circular motion. The same effect can be achieved with special rings that you can buy at the chemist's. You can store these bags filled with gel in the freezer or deep-freeze compartment of your fridge.

Compresses with teabags are also helpful. Pour a little hot water over two bags of standard black or camomile teabags. Let the bags cool down and place them over the eyelids for ten minutes. In future, think about keeping your used teabags for eye compresses! Eye gels with natural substances such as algae, horse chestnut, hamamelis or ginkgo have a revitalising effect. These are gently dabbed into the area around the eyes.

To relieve the connective tissue, you should cut down on your alcohol consumption, because most alcoholic beverages retain water in the tissues; beer, on the other hand, has a diuretic effect. Of course, mild natural diuretics such as tea made from birch leaves or nettles are much more healthy, but green tea and pu-erh tea also help to get rid of excess water. A glass of wine does no harm either, on the contrary – red wine is rich in antioxidants.

Dark rings under the eyes are often a telltale sign of a long night or an exhausting day at work. Even very pronounced rings will fade if you put some cool milk curds on them and let this take effect for 20 to 30 minutes. Another proven remedy for these unsightly rings are

raw grated potatoes. Simply place them on top of your closed eyes, lie back and let them take effect – but for no longer than three to five minutes.

People suffering from rings under their eyes should help the body work on this problem from the inside by chewing a few stalks of parsley every morning on an empty stomach.

Lines around the eyes are commonly known as crow's feet – not a very flattering name. However, they can be somewhat alleviated by compresses. You could perhaps try this household remedy: pour a cup of boiling water over five cloves and allow to draw for ten minutes in a covered container. Once the extract has cooled down, dab it onto the affected eye area with a cotton wool pad. You will see fast results with the latest preparations such as *biogyne lift patch* or the *anti-wrinkle plaster*.

COUPEROSIS: TRY NOT TO PROVOKE IT

Couperosis is a great problem for many women. Fine capillary vessels run through the skin; their diameter is so small that the red corpuscles are just able to pass through. This causes a capillary problem which manifests itself as a red "network", usually on the most exposed parts of the face such as the nose, cheeks or chin. However, this little blemish can become serious and can take the inflammatory form of acne rosacea. Possible causes of this skin problem are an innate weakness of the connective tissue and labile vascular walls. One clear sign that you are prone to couperosis is when you get rosy cheeks after taking a hot drink or after drinking alcohol, but also when it is very cold outside. You can also test your level of sensitivity by stretching your facial skin between your fingers. If the capillaries can be clearly seen, this is a sign that you could tend towards couperosis.

If you suffer from couperosis, you should avoid hot baths and saunas.

If you have a problem with couperosis, you must try to avoid everything that causes excess blood to flow through your skin. The list of forbidden substances includes alcohol-based facial lotions, rough-grained peeling mixtures, facial masks that dry on the skin and facial steam baths. When out in the sun, you must protect the affected parts of the skin with a sun cream with a high sun protection factor and an infrared filter. You should also protect your skin against extreme cold and biting winds with a cold weather protection cream.

The problem should be treated externally and internally at the same time. Care products, such as those from the Couperosal range, treat the skin from the outside, while you could try to regulate the inner fluid circulation with algae drinks and a mixture of valuable flavanoids, antioxidants and vitamins (angiobianes).

Wrinkles at an Early Age? No Need to Panic!

Those of us who have dry skin will unfortunately have to reckon with wrinkles at an early age. Lengthy periods of sunbathing can also avenge themselves in this way; skin specialists refer to this process as photo-aging. When wrinkles form, the skin loses its elasticity and natural moisture. With the right care, you will be able to delay this wrinkle formation. Skin smoothening masks and ampoules are like little energy injections, which almost instantaneously make wrinkles smaller, finer and almost invisible. These days, numerous anti-aging products provide help, and many of them are very effective indeed. It is up to the individual whether to use additional oxygen or vegetable nutrients to bring about that extra degree of success. Fine lines are flattened, the complexion appears fresher and on the whole you will find that your skin is much smoother.

Smoking has a negative effect on the metabolism and especially on the skin, because nicotine is an intensive vascular toxin. The carcinogenic tar forms a slag which the body disposes of in the connective tissue, once the fatty tissue can no longer serve this purpose. The skin appears grey, sallow and wrinkly. Of course it is better to stop smoking completely. However, if you are unable to do this you must support your skin, for example, with antioxidant vitamins and active ingredients from plants, especially those containing vitamin C – you can take up to 100 mg of this substance per day, assuming your GP has no resevations. Simple household remedies can also help: dab your face regularly with freshly pressed carrot juice – or grate an apple very finely and mix it with a tablespoon of honey. Apply this mixture like a facial mask and allow it to work in for 20 minutes. Then rinse it off with lukewarm water.

For a really efficient, professional treatment of wrinkles, you should consult your beautician. Besides providing you with nutritional advice and special ampoule treatments, beauticians will be able to help with special algae-based masks and anti-wrinkle plasters. Other methods of treatment are ultrasound and Iontophoresis.

Open Pores:
Tips for a Smooth Complexion

Having open-pored skin does not really have to mean that the pores are more open or rougher than normal. Actually the only portion that is more open is the visible part, the so-called pore outlet, because the callous skin at this point is swollen with sebum and moisture. This is why open-pored skin as a rule has an oily, shiny appearance.

The most important tip in caring for open-pored skin is to undergo peeling more often than with normal skin, perhaps twice a week, but less often in winter. When peeling oily skin, do not rub it too hard; simply massage the skin gently.

A marine mud and alumina facial mask applied twice a week will provide additional help. Another thing that may be worth trying is a regular papaya application. To make this, remove the fruit from its skin and puree it together with four tablespoons of pouring cream, then apply the mixture to the affected areas of the skin. Allow this to work in for thirty minutes and then rinse off with lukewarm water.

For care during the course of the day, you could use a cream containing fruit acid. These creams more or less constantly peel the skin and thus make it softer.

Stress Spots:
Don't Let Them Make You Nervous!

As a rule these are caused by a stressed-out nervous system and a certain degree of weakness in the vascular system. Some people break out into a sweat when they become tense and nervous and some suffer from stomach cramps, while others get red spots on their face. Therefore, the care must be aimed at dulling the sensitivity of the nerves and also boosting the blood circulation.

The following tricks can help you to handle the problem. First of all do without thick covering make-up and choose instead light, fresh products. Avoid stimulants such as coffee, tea and alcohol if you are serious about preventing stress spots appearing on your face.

Other facial spots – such as those caused by pigment problems – can be treated with skin care creams. Dab them regularly with a mixture of onion juice and cider vinegar in a ratio of 1:2 and you will soon find that they fade dramatically.

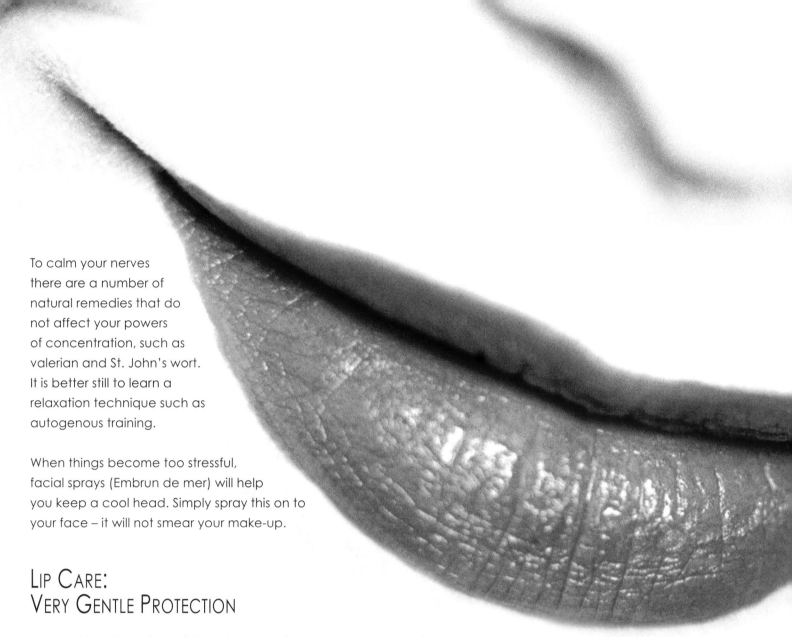

To calm your nerves there are a number of natural remedies that do not affect your powers of concentration, such as valerian and St. John's wort. It is better still to learn a relaxation technique such as autogenous training.

When things become too stressful, facial sprays (Embrun de mer) will help you keep a cool head. Simply spray this on to your face – it will not smear your make-up.

LIP CARE: VERY GENTLE PROTECTION

We would prefer to have full and luscious lips, but all too often things are usually quite different: they are cracked, pale and taut. Our lips are exceptionally sensitive, but in spite of this they are forced to face the wind and rain beside having to withstand intensive sunlight, freezing cold, overheated rooms and hot spices.

Dry, cracked lips need oil and moisture. It is best to care for them regularly with lip pomade. Why not try this home-made recipe for dry lips? Mix equal portions of milk curds and honey. Apply the paste to your lips and allow it to work in for half an hour. The best way to treat cracked lips is to smear them with thickened cream or unsalted butter.

Lip herpes is more of a medical ailment, but nevertheless it is also a cosmetic problem. Those of us who carry the virus around with us – in fact most

1 teaspoon beeswax granules
4 teaspoons jojoba oil
¹/₂ teaspoon liquid honey
1 drop pure essential rose oil

people – can suffer an outbreak every now and then; this can be caused by intensive sun, stress or feverish infections. You can alleviate this by applying an extract of rudbeckia and a drop of St. John's wort – or lemon balm, which is regarded as being the best cure. Severe itching can be alleviated with a few drops of tea tree oil.

Mix your own lip balsam à la rose. Melt the beeswax, jojoba oil and honey in a water bath, stirring intensively; then remove the pot from the heat and stir in the rose oil. Pour the balsam into a glass jar that can be sealed hermetically. Massage your lips with this mixture several times a day. When you take a portion of balsam from the jar, only do this with a spatula to prevent the mixture becoming contaminated.

PIMPLES, BLACKHEADS AND WHITEHEADS

There is no completely foolproof way to get rid of pimples and blackheads; but there are plenty ways to treat them.

Try not to squeeze pimples and blackheads – the germs on your fingers could otherwise get into the skin and make matters much worse. Young people especially are plagued by this problem, but also older people with oily and impure skin.

A facial steam bath is still the best way to get rid of skin impurities. The hot steam causes the pores to open slightly and the hard sebum, which blocks the pores, is dissolved. It is good to add disinfectant additives to such a steam bath, like camomile, marigold petals, sage or thyme. Even eight tablespoons of salt added to 2 litres (4 pints) of hot water will have a good cleansing effect. After the steam bath, wrap cellular cloths around your fingertips and squeeze the individual blackheads out from below without too much pressure. The effects of the steam bath or a hot compress can be intensified three to four times a week by applying a deep cleansing cream, for example our natural relaxation mask.

¹/₄ teaspoon green alumina
¹/₂ teaspoon ground almond powder
¹/₄ teaspoon oatmeal powder
3 tablespoons rose water
1 drop essential camomile oil
6 drops wheatgerm oil

In a glass bowl mix alumina, almond and oat flake powder. Place rose water, camomile oil and wheatgerm oil in a small pot and heat this mixture carefully, then allow it to cool. The next step is to add 5–10 ml (¹/₆–¹/₃ oz) of the liquid to the dry mixture and stir this until you have a homogeneous paste. Apply this in a thin layer to your face, neck and décolletage; leave the eyes free. Allow the mask to work in for ten minutes. Then dip two cotton wool pads in the remaining rose water mixture and use these as an eye compress. Remove the mask with mineral water.

Tea tree oil is an effective natural substance. Either a few drops are added to the water used to wash your face or else the individual blackheads or pimples are dabbed with some oil on a cotton wool tip. You could also try the following recipe: before going to bed, apply a mixture of equal parts of honey and pollard to the affected areas of skin. The next morning, rinse the mask off with lukewarm water.

BARE YOUR TEETH: TIPS FOR A SPARKLING SMILE

Dental care is an important part of personal hygiene – not to mention the cosmetic benefit. After all, you can only smile brightly at people if you are confident about the appearance of your teeth.

You get beautiful teeth by brushing them – for example with warm sage tea. This is also good for strengthening the gums. You can also whiten your teeth by brushing them with salt instead of toothpaste. And of course, strawberries taste much better than toothpaste: place a mashed strawberry on your toothbrush and clean your teeth with it. However, these time-honoured household recipes should only be used as a supplement to conventional dental care. It is important to use a high-quality toothpaste regularly; ask your dentist what he or she would recommend.

Tea drinkers in particular suffer from stained teeth. If you find that this is a problem, rinse your mouth with a teaspoon of cider vinegar after brushing your teeth; make quite sure that the vinegar gets in all the gaps. Having healthy teeth does not necessarily mean that you have pleasant smelling breath. Eating a fresh apple is a good way to combat bad breath – also before you go to bed as a preventive measure. If, in addition to this, you chew a sprig of parsley in the morning, your bad breath problems will soon be a thing of the past. A few grains of aniseed are a good way to get rid of the smell of garlic from your breath.

BEAUTIFUL, HEALTHY HAIR

Healthy hair is of course the most important prerequisite for a lovely hairstyle. Unfortunately however, many people do not give enough attention to their hair. This is a grave mistake, as the condition of our hair provides an insight into our physical and mental state. First of all your diet must be right so that your hair stays strong and healthy. Vitamins, minerals and trace elements are important for its structure and appearance. Deficiency symptoms in this area avenge themselves in the look of your hair: it appears lifeless and dull, is thin and tends to split easily. In some cases, hair loss can be attributed to nutritional causes.

HAIR PROBLEMS

Keratin, an elastic protein, accounts for ninety percent of our hair substance; the rest is made up of various minerals and moisture. The living part is the root, also called the hair follicle. This is where the most effective care and treatment should be applied, as hair has neither enzymes nor a metabolism like the skin, for instance. It can only be nourished via the blood circulation. Protein constituents, amino acids, minerals, trace elements, vitamins and polyunsaturated fatty acids are absorbed by the root, where they normally promote hair growth thanks to a healthy daily diet or with the assistance of nutrition supplements.

The outer, visible part of a hair consists of three layers. We have to take special care of the outer layer, the cuticle. Its tissue particles, arranged like

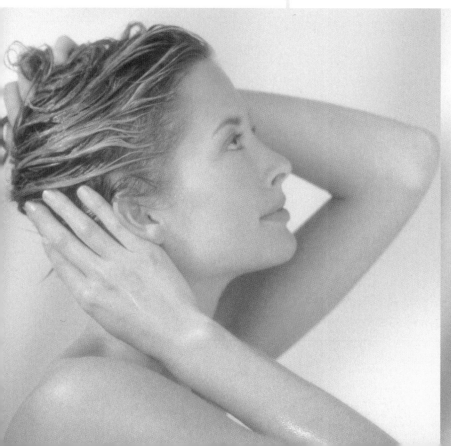
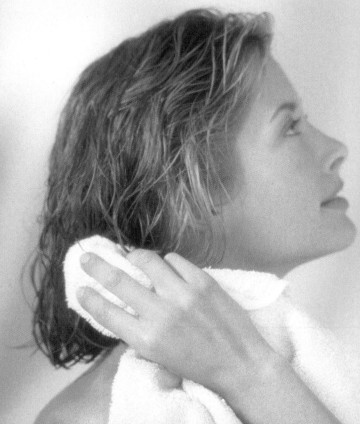

tiles on a roof, are the hair's protection and they should lie flat. If they are damaged by chemicals or high temperature, for instance, the hair becomes rough, lifeless, brittle and dull. Below the cuticle is the cortex, which is responsible for the hair's elasticity, strength and the even distribution of the pigment melanin. The third, inner layer, the medulla, supplies nutrients to the cortex and cuticle. Another substance that plays a part in the health and appearance of the hair is the sebum, which is secreted in the skin's sebaceous glands and in the hair roots. This ensures that the outer flaky layer lies flat and smooth and is closed up, so that it cannot dry out. If the sebaceous glands fail to produce sufficient sebum, the hair dries out and can become brittle.

Excess production of sebum is the cause of greasy, straggly and heavy hair. If you have dry hair and a greasy scalp (seborrhoea), it is necessary to attack the problem on two fronts. As a rule, the greasy root is caused by a hormonal imbalance and can be treated by a gynaecologist.

Brittle hair and split ends are not just a problem for people with long hair. Even short hair can have limited strength. Shampooing your hair too often, the chemical effects of dying or toning or the effects or a perm can be the cause of this problem, as can intensive sun or insufficient nutrition of the hair roots.

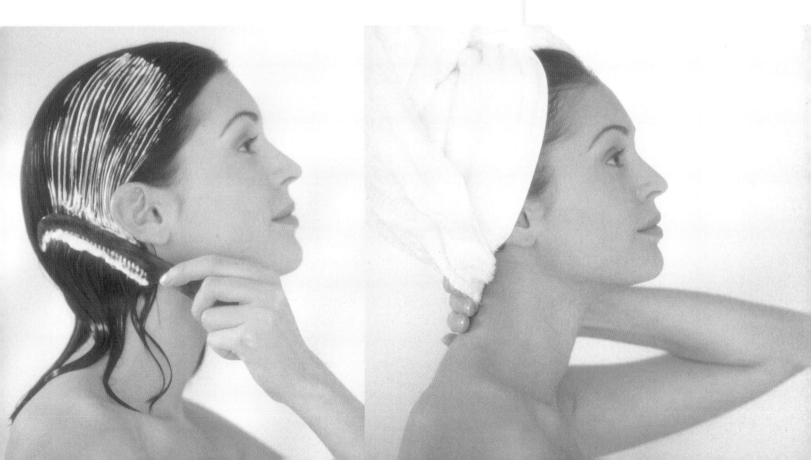

Hair loss can be caused by quite a number of factors: it can be hereditary or the result of an illness, a medication or a therapy. In any case, it is important that you have the problem examined by a hair expert; and in more serious cases, it is better to consult a dermatologist.

Optimum Hair Care

Don't use just any old shampoo; remember that hair care begins with choosing the right product to suit your hair. Choose neutral or weak acidic preparations with a pH of between 5 and 7. In this way you will not be risking any structural changes to the flaky layer. Water with a pH above seven makes your hair start to swell up! Perm, blonding and dying products are quite strongly alkaline, with a pH of as much as 8 to 11.

Remember the following rules when washing your hair. First remove all hair spray and dirt particles with a soft brush; then wash the comb and brush immediately. Read the instructions on the shampoo bottle carefully: different shampoos remain on your hair for different lengths of time. Take these instructions seriously.

Change your shampoo often to ensure that your hair is provided with the maximum active ingredients. And remember: good shampoos clean your hair without producing a crown of foam on top of your head.

Wash your hair under lukewarm water, moving your fingertips in a gentle circular motion. Be especially thorough at the hairline to remove cream and make-up residues. Rinse the shampoo from your hair thoroughly without tugging at it; wet hair splits more easily. Always use a wide-toothed comb to comb your hair while it is wet.

When drying your hair with a hairdrier, always hold it at least 12 cm (about 5 inches) from your head to prevent your hair from overheating and getting tangled.

In order to help the scaly outer layer of your hair close again, you should treat your hair with an acid rinse, for example a tablespoonful of cider vinegar or the juice of half a lemon. If the hair is permed or you have split ends, a hair conditioner (for instance *Baume Demêlant*) is an absolute must, as otherwise you would tug your hair too much with the comb, which could in turn damage the individual hairs over their entire length.

A head massage is recommended for stimulating the circulation and thus enhancing the supply of oxygen and nutrition to the hair follicles. Massage towards the middle of your head, without too much pressure. Do not rub your scalp. You should also use a high-quality hair tonic. The mechanical effects of the massage can be supported internally with an algae drink. The aqueous extract of the alga *delesseria sanguinea* is especially suitable for the hair roots as a stimulant for cell growth.

RINSES, PACKS AND OIL BATHS

Depending on how much time you want to spend and on the condition of your hair, you can choose between a simple herb rinse, an intensive rinse for frayed and unruly hair (a must for chemically treated and frequently styled hair), a structuring spray as a protection against electrostatic charging, and warm oil baths (be careful with water-soluble oils or solutising agents, as you will then have to shampoo your hair afterwards if you do not want it to tangle). Besides this, repair foam for split ends is available: in this case a microscopically fine layer of smoothing film is left on the freshly washed hair. You can achieve the same effect with a pack for permed and dyed hair: the substances remain in the hair, where they cover the brittle parts. Research has provided us with valuable new products; nevertheless, natural cosmetics are no less effective than they were in our grandmother's day.

For greasy hair, a beer rinse with 250 ml ($^1/_2$ pint) of any light beer, before putting curlers in, can be used as a substitute for a setting lotion. There are numerous reasonably priced herbal rinses readily available, including henna, which is probably the best known plant extract. This gives dark hair a warm, reddish sheen, while lighter hair can turn titian red. Henna is not especially suitable for white or blonde hair. In any case, you should make a test with henna before applying it to all of your hair and then adhere closely to the manufacturer's instructions.

NATURAL RECIPES FOR YOUR HAIR

There is a simple household recipe which helps combat dandruff in dry or normal hair. Mix olive oil and diluted rosemary oil with two drops of essential camomile oil and one drop of essential lavender oil. Add two capsules of vitamin E or evening primrose oil. Keep this mixture in dark-coloured

20 ml ($^2/_3$ oz) native olive oil from the first press
10 ml ($^1/_3$ oz) diluted water-soluble rosemary oil
2 drops essential camomile oil
1 drop essential lavender oil
2 capsules vitamin E or evening primrose oil

bottles. This recipe is sufficient for two treatments per week after a mild shampoo. Carefully massage the solution into your scalp, strand by strand. Also apply some of the solution to the body of the hair itself. Allow the mixture to work in for about thirty minutes under a shower cap, then rinse it out with a mild shampoo.

15 ml (¹/₂ oz) cider vinegar
4 drops essential rosemary oil
2 drops essential lavender oil
200 ml (7 oz) distilled water

Use cider vinegar to make a lotion for normal hair or for hair that tends to be on the oily side. Once you have added the essential oils, fill the solution into a dark bottle. Shake the mixture vigorously, add the distilled water and then shake it again. Treat your hair with this mixture once or twice every week or, if your hair is greasy, three times a week.

2 eggs
2 teaspoons liquid honey
3–4 teaspoons thistle oil,
alternatively:
2 tablespoons avocado oil
1 tablespoon castor oil
1 egg

This preliminary shampoo used before your regular shampoo is especially recommended for dry hair with or without split ends. Depending on the length of your hair, this mixture is sufficient for one or two applications. Mix honey and oil together and then add the eggs. Massage this cocktail into your hair, cover with a pre-warmed terry towelling cap or a shower cap and allow the mixture to soak in for 30 minutes. Then wash it out with a mild shampoo. You can also vary this recipe and compose a pre-shampoo from an egg, avocado oil and castor oil.

Also available are natural shampoos made from algae. *Algologie Shampooing aux Algues* for normal hair contains micro-fine chopped algae (fucus vesiculus), tensio-active substances, silk proteins and essential lavender oil. By using this shampoo you are providing your hair with all the active ingredients of the ocean's elemental power. If you have oily hair, use *Algologie Shampooing au Ghassoul*, which has an oil-absorbing effect due to the balancing influence of African alumina. *Algologie Shampooing au Monoi* is especially suitable for fine and dry hair, as it cleanses and nourishes the hair at the same time, counteracts dehydration and gives it a silky sheen.

Algae extracts can be used
for hair problems of all kinds. This can
be supported by an internal hair
cure with Algae-Vital capsules or an
algae drink.

Monoi oil is obtained from grated coconut and macerated with costly flower petals. This process produces exceptionally high-quality oil that makes the skin soft and supple. Monoi is the ideal product for dry hair and split ends. It is used in both shampoos and hair packs together with algae. Before giving yourself this treatment, you should carefully brush your hair with a natural bristle brush to remove dirt particles and hair lacquer, and then apply the first oil pack. Allow it to work in for 15 minutes under a warm terry towelling compress, and then rinse it out with monoi shampoo – twice if necessary.

It is also important that you wash your hair correctly. Place a nut-sized portion of shampoo on your wet hands and massage it into your hair intensively, but without rubbing. Allow it to work in for about two minutes and then thoroughly rinse it out. You can repeat this procedure if necessary. By "thoroughly" rinsing, we mean that the shampooed hair must be rinsed seven to nine times with clear water. If your hair is difficult to comb, it is important to apply some hair conditioner after shampooing, for example *Baume Démêlant*. Massage this into your hair and then rinse it out thoroughly.

If your scalp is dry, it is recommended that you use a post-shampoo. For one to two applications, mash half a ripe avocado together with a teaspoonful of avocado oil and an egg yolk and beat this mixture with an egg whisk. Massage it into your scalp and rinse it out with warm water after ten minutes.

$^1/_2$ ripe avocado
1 teaspoon avocado oil
1 egg yolk

If you have oily, fine hair, make a post-shampoo from five tablespoons of natural yoghurt and an egg. Massage this into your scalp and rinse it out again after five to ten minutes.

5 tablespoons natural yoghurt
1 egg

You can prepare an effective natural pack for grey hair. Place two tablespoons of dried sage and one tablespoon of Indian tea in a teapot and fill it with boiling water. Put the lid on the pot and allow to brew for ten minutes. Then mix the brew with kaolin powder to form a paste and spread this over your hair; then rinse the pack out of your hair again after about 20 minutes.

2 tablespoons dried sage
1 tablespoon Indian tea
5 tablespoons kaolin
500 ml (1 pint) water

In order to protect your hair from the sun's rays, chlorine from the swimming pool or the effects of a long period of bathing in the sea, massage a mixture of three teaspoons of coconut oil and four drops of pure essential ylang-ylang oil into your scalp and hair. This composition is also ideal for a 30-minute pack for tired and dull hair. A mild shampoo is recommended afterwards.

3 teaspoons coconut oil
4 drops essential ylang-ylang oil

You should always use a high-quality hair tonic after shampooing, for example Algae-Vital hair tonic R or AF. This is applied to the scalp and massaged in with the fingertips, using a circular motion. Algae-Vital hair tonic can be used every day – also as a preventive measure against hair loss in men. As the costly natural active ingredients are not filtered out during manufacture, you should always shake the bottle thoroughly before using this tonic.

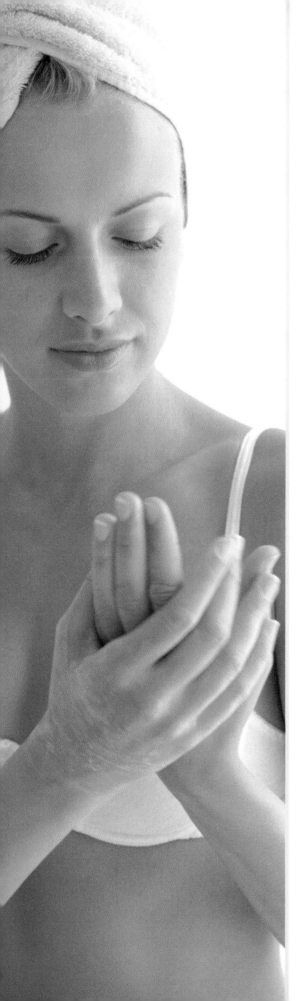

The more damaged, porous and dry your hair is, the greater its nutrient requirements will be; in such cases, you will have to determine the dosage yourself depending on the condition of your hair. You can use a moist, warm terry towel or a plastic shower cap to ensure that the active ingredients penetrate more deeply. Before thoroughly rinsing your hair with lukewarm water, begin with just a little water. Finally, dry your hair thoroughly and comb it out with a wooden or tortoiseshell comb (and not with a synthetic comb, as this would cause your hair to charge electrostatically). Put some Algae-Vital hair tonic in an eggcup or a liqueur glass and use cotton wool to apply this high-quality product to the roots, strand by strand.

However, you should bear in mind that an external treatment is seldom sufficient to obtain or keep beautiful healthy hair; a balanced diet is very important. You can also improve the quality of your hair by taking some alumina orally. Alumina is regarded as a cosmetic for both internal and external application. This valuable mineral product, which is not subjected to detrimental environmental influences as it comes from deep down in the earth, is so significant for an inner treatment because of its high concentration of silica salts (which are important for the connective tissue and blood vessels). Alumina also contains magnesium, iron and other organic minerals and trace elements. By taking three to six alumina capsules each day with plenty of fluid, you will soon get your metabolism back in balance.

Your Hands: Care Makes Them Beautiful

Our hands are our most important tools, but in spite of this we often do not take enough care of them. The first signs of aging can often be seen on a person's hands, and yet few people make sufficient effort to alleviate these signs. After all, you can't get a hand-lift in the same way as a face-lift. It is therefore important to take good care of your hands as long as they are still fresh and young. The first and most important consideration in hand care is that they should be cleaned properly. Always use mild soap to wash your hands; and never forget to cream them after each wash. They should also be given a special treatment once a week. This could be as follows:

Clean your hands with a mild peeling product, the same as you use for your face. Especially good for this purpose are enzyme packs, which only have to be mixed with water. A pack that pampers tired facial skin is also good for stressed hands.

You can treat rough skin, also on your forearms, with a special hand oil that can easily be prepared at home – by the way, this recipe is also good for tired computer hands! Mix a teaspoonful each of diluted East Indian geranium oil and sweet almond oil with a drop each of pure essential camomile oil and lavender oil.

1 teaspoon diluted East Indian geranium oil
1 teaspoon sweet almond oil
1 drop essential camomile oil
1 drop essential lavender oil

At this point we would like to recommend a special protective cream for your hands. It is admittedly somewhat more complicated and time-consuming to prepare, but as you will see, it is well worth the effort. Melt 15 g ($^1/_2$ oz) of grated beeswax in a water bath and add a teaspoon of honey and 160 ml ($5^1/_2$ oz) of sweet almond oil. Add the contents of four capsules of evening primrose oil to this molten mass. Then slowly add the distilled water – at first just in drops. Use a mixing spoon or a whisk to obtain a homogeneous mixture. For the sake of hygiene, it is important that the vessels and mixing tools are first disinfected with alcohol (70 percent). Once you have added two teaspoons of distilled water to the mixture, immediately remove it from the heat and gradually add the rest of the water. Finally, while still stirring, add the essential oils – five drops each of East Indian geranium oil, orange blossom oil and lavender oil. Stir this fragrant mixture until it thickens, then immediately pour it into a sterile glass jar. You should make sure to attach a label to the jar stating when its contents were made, as this cream can only be used for about three months at the most.

15 g ($^1/_2$ oz) beeswax, grated
1 teaspoon liquid honey
160 ml ($5^1/_2$ oz) sweet almond oil
4 capsules evening primrose oil
350 ml (12 oz) distilled water
5 drops essential East Indian geranium oil
5 drops essential orange blossom oil
5 drops essential lavender oil

Apply this cream to your hands every evening before going to bed, then put on a pair of old leather gloves. Also take a capsule of borage and fish oil. In this way, the treatment will be effective both externally and internally.

Dry hands? – no problem. Your dry hands and cracked skin will really appreciate a hot oil bath each week. Prepare your bath with East Indian geranium oil and borage oil. It is very important that you wear leather gloves overnight.

Red hands? – no problem. Warm milk baths – twice a week – soon put an end to unsightly redness.

Sweaty hands? – no problem. A moist handshake is dubious pleasure. But you can do something about sweaty hands: washing with spirit of camphor will often help.

Spotty hands? – no problem. Hands that work hard seldom appear clean and cared for. Housework in particular leaves telltale signs. Hands that appear dirty after peeling potatoes are best cleaned by rubbing them with vinegar or lemon juice. Nicotine stains become less obvious if they are rubbed with some icing sugar mixed with lemon juice. But the best way of caring for your hands is to wear gloves – which is why you should get into this habit for certain kitchen tasks.

Smelly hands? – no problem. Kitchen smells tend to adhere to your hands, especially if you have been chopping vegetables, and quite often remain there for some time. If you want to chop onions, for instance, you should rub some olive oil into your hands beforehand, and then they will not absorb the smell. Moist salt also helps against the smell of onion and fish – however, this only takes effect afterwards.

HEALTHY FINGERNAILS: A MUST FOR BEAUTIFUL HANDS

Firm, resilient fingernails are an important prerequisite for beautiful hands. But it is no easy matter to keep nails healthy and strong. They are very susceptible to environmental effects, incorrect treatment and faulty nutrition. Healthy nails require constant care. For instance, they are particularly sensitive in winter. As hard nails are also dry, they respond well to some moisture. Choose a hand cream that is enriched with natural oils, for example sweet almond oil. Even varnished nails should be rubbed with this twice daily.

If you neglect to apply a protective base varnish nail blemishes are only to be expected. These unsightly yellow spots can be removed with a nail peeling, in the process of which the top layer of nail is scrubbed off.

The most common problem with fingernails is that they become brittle. This happens when the sealing substance between the individual nail layers is damaged. The following nail pack can solve this problem. Mix two teaspoonfuls of olive oil with two teaspoonfuls of lecithin powder into a paste and massage some of this on to your nails and the nail bed. Then apply the rest thickly and rinse it off with lukewarm water after half an hour. You can also buy nail packs that contain structuring substances. Yeast also helps brittle nails, but it is only effective when used over an extended period.

The area surrounding your nails must also be treated with particuar care. You should avoid cutting off cuticles; push them back instead with a wooden tool. If the cuticles are cracked and dry you can treat them with warm oil baths containing almond or olive oil.

Making your own special oil for the nails and cuticles is quite a simple matter: put 100 ml (about $3^1/_2$ oz) of almond oil, 50 ml ($1^2/_3$ oz) of castor oil and 50 ml ($1^2/_3$ oz) of avocado oil together with two drops of bitter almond oil and 50 g ($1^2/_3$ oz) of vaseline into an ovenproof receptacle and heat this mixture in a water bath. When the vaseline has melted and combined with the oils, allow the mass to cool and pour into a clean receptacle. Rub this mixture into your fingers regularly.

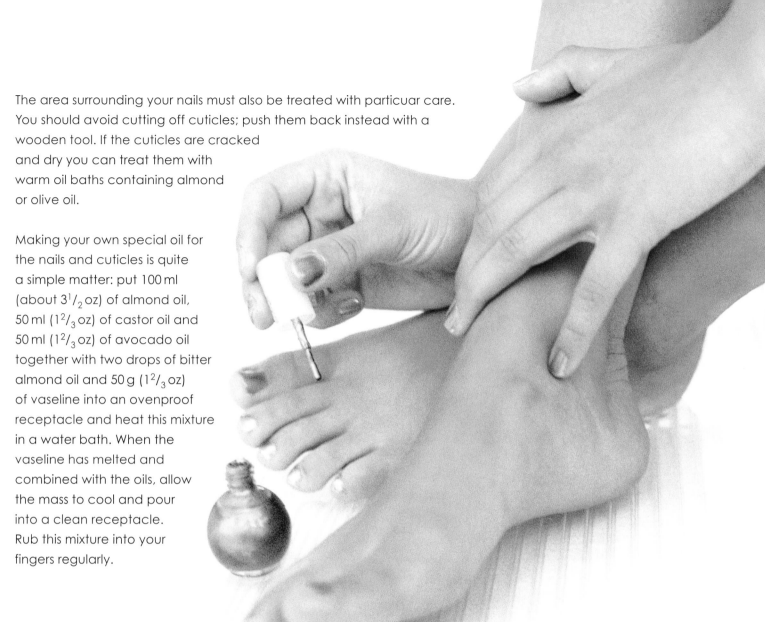

Your Feet

With the feet and toenails the situation is similar to the hands and fingernails: they are all too frequently neglected. If you regularly visit a podiatrist, your feet will certainly thank your for it. However, you can care for your feet yourself – 20 minutes a week are quite sufficient.

The most common cause of unsightly feet are shoes that are too tight. Pressure points can cause calluses, painful blisters, annoying corns and onchytis. Our feet are always more swollen in the afternoon than in the morning. So the most suitable time to buy shoes is any time after about 4 o'clock in the afternoon.

When choosing shoes, comfort should take priority over fashion, even if most people will not like to hear this. By the way, it is not true that high heels automatically cause foot and back problems. On the contrary – by alternating between high heels and flat shoes, you are training your muscles.

After a warm – if possible alkaline – footbath, which should take around a qurater of an hour, smoothen the rough areas with pumice stone or a callus rasp. Cut soft toenails with scissors; clippers are better for harder nails. Give your nails that finishing touch with a crystal file (diamond, sapphire or ceramic). Then push the cuticles back into place with a wooden tool.

One of the most common problems with toenails are grooves, which can be the sign of a vitamin deficiency or an infection. Consult your dermatologist to get to the root of the problem and find a possible cure. Once the cause has been discovered and redressed, the grooves can be smoothend with a polishing file until the toenails grow back naturally.

Just as with fingernails, many people suffer from brittle and cracked toenails. To solve this problem, you should treat your toes to a foot mask every now and then. You don't need any expensive accessories; all you have to do is massage your toes and nails with a special massage oil mixture – plus 5 ml ($^1/_6$ oz) of lemon grass oil, one drop of geranium oil and two drops of santal oil – before going to bed and then cover your feet with cotton socks for the night. The next morning, you will find that your feet are soft and smooth.

FOOTBATHS ALLEVIATE PROBLEMS

To prepare your feet for this treatment, add a few drops of essential lavender or almond oil to your footbath.

It is quite normal to have swollen feet and tired legs after an exhausting day at work. But footbaths can help make them fit again: peppermint, for instance, regenerates tired feet in next to no time. Pour 1 litre (2 pints) of boiling water over a handful of peppermint leaves and allow this mixture to brew for 15 minutes. Then strain off the liquid and bathe your feet in it for ten minutes.

Cider vinegar is effective in combating sweaty feet. You can get rid of unpleasant smells by regularly bathing your feet in a mixture of water and cider vinegar (proportion 1:2). If used daily, the cider vinegar mixed with warm water will begin to take effect after just one week.

This recipe helps against calluses on the feet: pour three teaspoons of cider vinegar into a dark-coloured 30 ml (1 oz) bottle and add two drops of essential santal oil. Then seal the bottle and shake vigorously to mix the ingredients. Finally, add 10 ml ($^1/_3$ oz) of diluted lemon grass oil and 5 ml ($^1/_6$ oz) of grapeseed oil. Shake the bottle once more. Store it in a cool dark place and use up the contents within two weeks. First bathe your feet for ten minutes in warm soapy water to soften the calluses. Then dry them and massage the above mixture into your feet. Repeat this procedure every day for two weeks.

Painful pressure points can also be made to disappear overnight, if you bathe your feet in a herbal or alkaline footbath each evening. Then heat some olive oil in a water bath and massage this into your feet. Wear socks in bed.

YOUR LEGS

Short skirts, tight shorts or dresses with seductive slits: for all of these, you need attractive legs. However, beautiful legs are not a godsend – they are the result of intensive care.

Most women are convinced that their legs do not comply with popular beauty standards. Too short or too long, to fat or too thin; for some, it is cellulitis, and for others it is phleboectasy that supposedly makes their legs so unsightly. The most common fear is cellulitis; this is a problem for around 80 percent of women. It is therefore understandable that research institutes and the cosmetic industry are constantly coming up with new preparations and methods of treatment. Admittedly, one should not always take all the promises at face value, as no miracle cure has yet been discovered that can make cellulitis disappear more or less overnight. There are many different causes for this disorder, such as blood circulation problems, changes in the hormonal balance, faulty nutrition or a lack of exercise.

One should be careful in diagnosing cellulitis. If you suspect that you suffer from this condition, it is best to consult an experienced beautician, who can form a reliable diagnosis on the basis of a discussion and a question-naire. A correct diagnosis is not just based on tests aimed at examining the

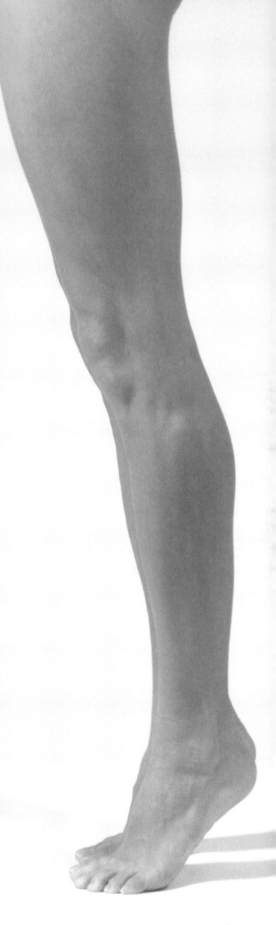

condition of the skin – "orange skin" tests and pinching tests – but also on information and the condition of the entire body. Is the digestive system in good condition? Can any hereditary factors be determined? Does the person have any other illnesses such as liver or kidney problems that could be responsible for the cell inflammation? Even spinal damage, weak connective tissue, leg problems, thrombosis or rheumatism of the soft tissue can play a role.

A reliable method of determining the extent of the cellulitis is echography. The patient lies down and the cellulite infiltrate is measured with the aid of an ultrasound sensor. If the fatty tissue is less than 15 mm (about $^5/_8$ inch) in thickness, local cosmetic measures are usually sufficient. However, if the fatty tissue is between 15 and 45 mm (about $^5/_8$ and $1^3/_4$ inches) thick, a more intensive internal and external treatment will be required. If the fatty tissue is thicker than 45 mm ($1^3/_4$ inches), a complicated holistic therapy will be necessary.

Regular exercise is another important factor in this treatment. Modern gyms have special exercises dedicated to the problem zones of the thighs and bottom. Besides this, anything that exercises your legs is good – for instance cycling, swimming, walking or skipping.

The most important consideration in ensuring successful treatment is that the therapy is started at an early stage. However, patience and discipline are required before the first signs of success become apparent; it is not something that sets in from one day to the next. The therapy is essentially aimed at stimulating the blood circulation, tightening the tissue and burning up fat. Algae have proved to be very effective in this connection: they are combined externally (in the form of algae baths, algae extracts, algae macerations, algae gels and algae packs) and internally. They tighten the tissue, bind moisture and burn up fat cells.

If you want to make sure you do not get cellulitis, you must pay attention to your weight. Modern radical diets are no use; the only way to stay slim is to adhere to a healthy, balanced diet and to understand how it works. For instance, this includes knowing that oxygen absorption and anoxaemia (oxygen deficiency) are mainly dependent on the properties of the fat cells and that burning up nutrients is an important part of the body's overall metabolism. It can be advisable to ask your GP for his or her advice if you believe that your fat metabolism is out of balance. Besides this, you should drink a lot, approximately 3 litres (6 pints) of still mineral water or fresh vegetable juice each day; of this, you should drink at least $^1/_4$ litre ($^1/_2$ pint) in the morning.

Dilated tiny veins in the legs are another very common problem. These take the form of a fine bluish network of veins, mainly in the thighs and ankles.

HOW TO REMOVE ANNOYING HAIR FROM YOUR LEGS

Hair on the legs is a cosmetic problem that simply will not go away, no matter how intensively you care for your legs. Which method you use to remove this annoying hair really depends on your sensitivity to pain and how long you expect the result to last. You can choose from the following methods:

Simply "cream" it away

The cream or foam hair removal products on the market work on the basis of active ingredients that rapidly dissolve the hair keratin below the surface of the skin. The paste can be removed with a spatula soon after it has been applied, and you will have smooth legs as a result. This procedure has to be repeated about once a week.

A quick shave

Wet or dry – the effect is the same. The advantage of shaving your legs is that it is quick and does not hurt. However, the disadvantage is that the hair grows back again within a few days and it is then rather stubbly.

Plucking

This is called epilation. Electric epilation devices pluck the hair from the skin with rotating pincers. The first time you do this it is a relatively painful procedure, because it pinches – but you will soon get used to it. The clear advantage of this method is that it takes three to four weeks for the fine hair to grow back again.

Traditional depilation

The traditional method of removing hair with wax is quite thorough, but rather painful. It feels as if a sticking plaster were being pulled from the skin. The simplest method is with cold wax. You can buy ready-made strips, which you place over the skin and then peel away. Warm wax, on the other hand, must be applied accurately to ensure that even the tiniest hairs are removed. It is important to press the wax in the direction of growth and to pull it off in the opposite direction. The advantage of this method is that your legs generally remain smooth for three to four weeks and the hair that then grows back is soft. However, as already mentioned, the treatment is rather unpleasant.

This can be caused by weak connective tissue, but it could also be a sign of a more serious vascular problem. In any case, it is advisable to have your legs examined by your GP, as purely cosmetic treatment should only be used in the case of a weakness in the surface connective tissue.

Alternating hot and cold showers on the legs can be a good form of gymnastics for the blood vessels. To do this, spray your legs with hot or cold water from bottom to top; always start on the outside of the leg and then continue on the inside. This treatment should only be carried out if you have no serious vein problems.

AN ATTRACTIVE BUST

For most women, an attractive bust is just as important as a well cared-for complexion. And still, most women are dissatisfied with what they have been given by nature. Too small or too large, too flabby or asymmetrical – the list of perceived faults is indeed long. While size can be corrected by surgery, weak tissue is something that you must treat yourself. The female breast consists mainly of soft fatty tissue, glandular tissue and connective tissue, all of which rest loosely on top of a large muscle. If this is not exercised occasionally, the breast becomes slack. Pregnancy, weak connective tissue, bad posture and long periods spent sunbathing all contribute to hanging breasts. Unfortunately, there is no cosmetic means of getting hanging breasts back in form, but there is a lot you can do beforehand to ensure that this situation does not arise in the first place, or at least that it is delayed.

CARE AND HOUSEHOLD REMEDIES

Special breast preparations improve the microcirculation in the tissue. They will not make your breasts larger, but they do ensure that the skin becomes firmer. Most of these products contain vitamins and minerals as well as special active anti-aging ingredients. Embrocations of fresh pineapple juice or a brew of alchemilla or ground coriander in honey are said to help. An insider tip is raw apple puree: grate two to three apples and apply the puree to both breasts. Allow this to work in for fifteen minutes and then rinse it off with cold water under the shower.

COOL AFFUSIONS AND SOFT BRUSHES

The skin of your décolletage holds your breasts like a natural bra. This can be seen clearly if you stretch your chin forwards – your breasts will lift slightly. That is also why it is so important to include the décolletage in all care measures. Cold affusions and treatment with ice cubes are a time-honoured remedy – and they do help. For instance, after showering you should spray your breasts with a weak stream of cold water. Treat both breasts in a clockwise direction. If you feel up to it, you can also rub them with an ice-cold flannel or with ice cubes. Another very effective method is to brush your breasts each evening with a soft brush. Massage in a circular motion, but avoid brushing your nipples.

A STRAIGHT BACK AND ISOMETRIC EXERCISES

Ensuring that you maintain a correct posture is half the secret of success. Chin up, shoulders back and chest out! Check your posture from time to time in the mirror. Exercising helps strengthen the large chest muscle. The ideal form of gymnastics are isometric exercises, which activate the muscles but hardly move the breasts themselves. A simple everyday exercise is the Indian greeting – press your hands flat against each other in front of your chest. Keep your forearms horizontal and your elbows raised. Now press the palms of your hands firmly against one another – hold the tension for ten seconds and then relax. Repeat this exercise sev-

You can combine breast care with your regular health checks. Examine your breasts with your fingertips once a month to make sure there are no lumps.

eral times. Another method of training the chest muscles is to practise dry swimming movements.

And now for a word on bras. Many women still apparently believe that wearing a bra relaxes the muscles and that it is better to do without one. In fact, exactly the opposite is true – the tissue needs support to stay firm. A well-fitting bra is therefore ideal for this purpose.

Your neck and décolletage also need a great deal of care and attention. After bathing, you should pay special attention to these parts of your body. Neck compresses are very good. Make a neck compress with borage oil or a mixture of equal parts of olive oil and almond oil; heat the oil in a water bath and then soak a gauze bandage in the mixture and wrap it around your neck. To enhance the effect of the heat, you could wrap some plastic film around the bandage and then cover it with a thin towel soaked in hot water.

A Firm Bottom

A really firm bottom has two main characteristics: taut muscles, which require constant exercise, and silky smooth skin, which needs intensive care.

Training the muscles in your bottom is relatively easy to fit into your day-to-day schedule. It is something that you can do almost anywhere. For example, you can exercise while sitting down: repeatedly tense the muscles in your bottom as if you were trying to hold a pencil between your buttocks, and then relax. Eight times in a row is sufficient. Another exercise is to lie on your back and place your heels on a chair. Now press your heels down against the chair for six seconds, without lifting your bottom from the floor. Also repeat this exercise eight times.

Another exercise that is good for a firm bottom is the catwalk. That is the way models walk when modelling clothes. This cat-like form of walking is done by moving your legs not parallel with one another but with a swing of the hip. This requires some practice, but it is a good form of exercise for your bottom. If you skip the lift and use the stairs more often, you will also be doing something to improve these muscles.

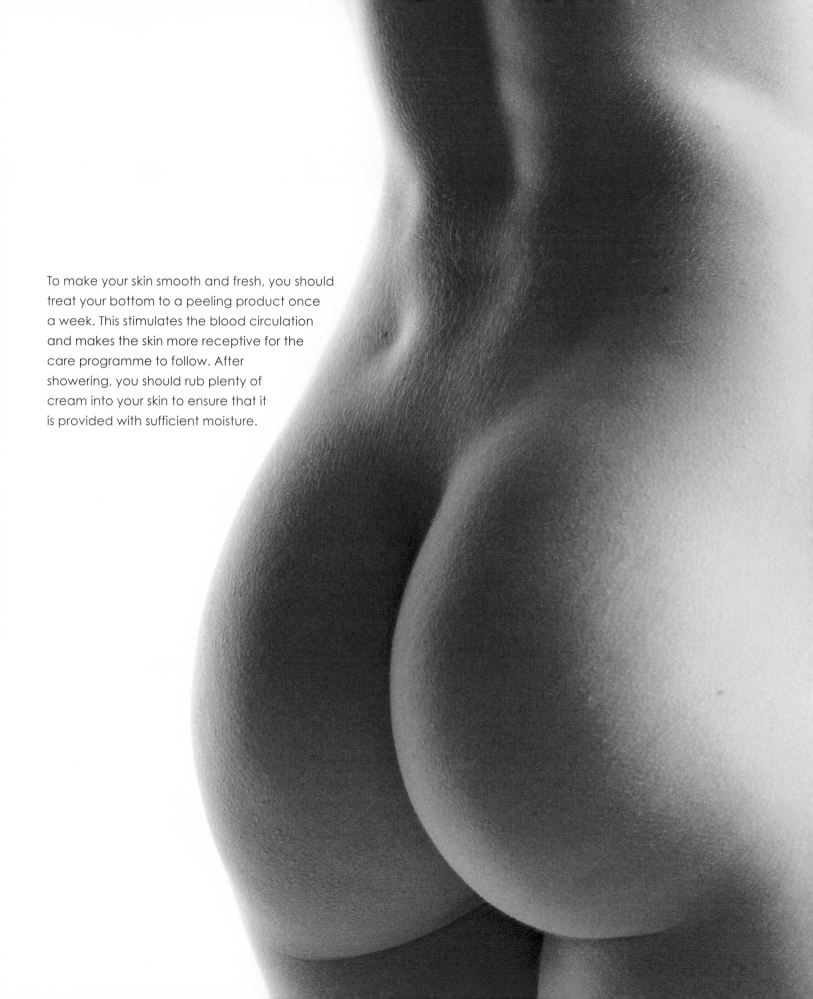

To make your skin smooth and fresh, you should treat your bottom to a peeling product once a week. This stimulates the blood circulation and makes the skin more receptive for the care programme to follow. After showering, you should rub plenty of cream into your skin to ensure that it is provided with sufficient moisture.

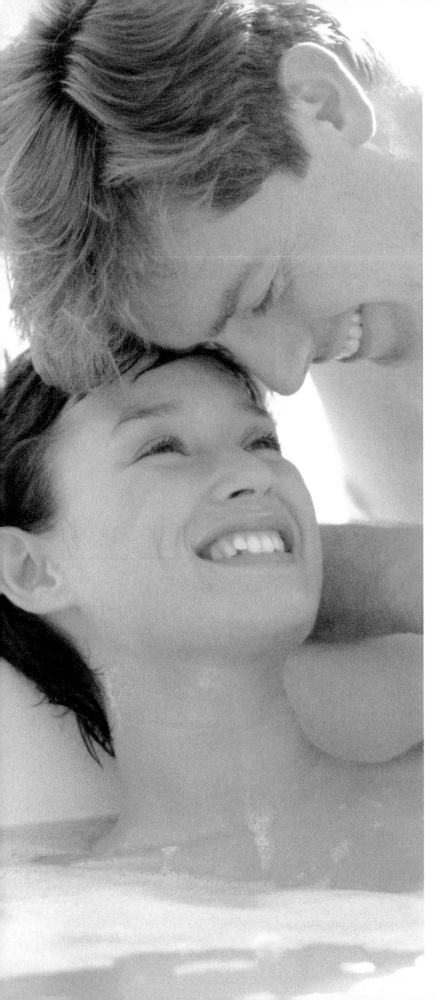

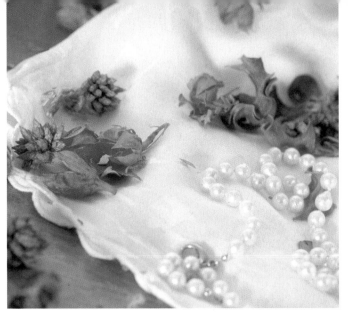

BATHING AND SHOWERING ARE A WAY OF WITHDRAWING INTO OURSELVES AND THOROUGHLY ENJOYING THE WONDERFUL FEELING THAT THE WATER GIVES US. IN THIS WAY, THE BODY GENERATES RENEWED VITALITY AND THE SOUL IS BALANCED AGAIN. SHARING THIS EXPERIENCE WITH A LOVED ONE AND PAMPERING ONE ANOTHER IS LIKE A PORTAL TO PARADISE. WITH THE MAGIC OF FRESH, CAPTIVATING AROMAS, THE WATER THAT SURROUNDS YOUR BODY AND THE BLISSFUL FEELING OF GENTLY TOUCHING ONE ANOTHER, A BATH TOGETHER CAN BECOME A CELEBRATION OF LOVE. BUT REMEMBER, EXPERIENCES SUCH AS THIS SHOULD BE PLANNED CAREFULLY AND WITH IMAGINATION.

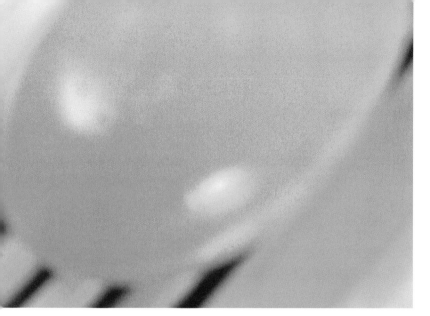
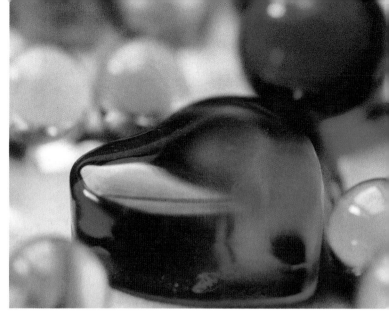

A Bath for Two

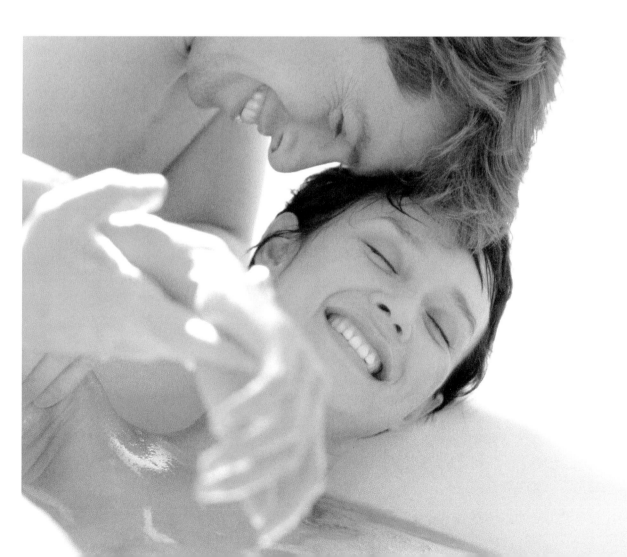

PRIVATE BATHING PLEASURES

Bathing and showering number among the most basic needs of every human being; after all, we all want to be clean. But bathing and showering can more than just fulfil a need for personal hygiene: they can amount to pleasure, wallowing in pleasant feelings, sinking into a condition that is somewhere between reality and the dreamworld, allowing yourself to float along wherever your dreams may take you.

Showering or bathing together might seem a little strange at first when one considers the usual domestic circumstances: who has such a spacious shower or bath that two adults can stand or sit in it together? It looks wonderful in films when the loving couple splashes around in the generously dimensioned bath that often is more like a miniature swimming pool, drinking champagne and celebrating their love. However, when one imagines these machinations in the bath at home, where there is often just enough room for one person with his or her knees drawn up – if two people were to share the bath one would have to bend oneself up like a pocket knife with the tap jammed uncomfortably into one's back – it is difficult to see anything positive in sharing a bath. How could that be particularly enjoyable?

Bathing in the bath or shower is an intimate matter: the opportunity to withdraw into yourself and think of no one else, to dedicate your thoughts to your own body, to touch it lovingly with a soapy sponge. Most people want to be left in peace when they are bathing. Children and pets should remain outside. Nothing that could disturb your train of thought should allowed into the bathroom. When relaxing in the luxuriant bath foam, you do not want to have to bother about what others think. The bath, the shower – both are a very personal experience, a decidedly egotistic pleasure.

But this is no argument against bathing with a loved one, an experience sought together. A bath for rheumatism – to take a prosaic example – is taken alone. This type of bath only fulfils a rudimentary purpose. Basically, it is similar to a taking the waters – it is a therapy. And on top of this, one is condemned to suffer the pain, the illness. No one would ever consider taking a rheumatism bath that smells strongly of menthol just for pleasure. Of course, it is by no means unpleasant – the warm water with the healing additives may even make you feel much better; and on top of this, the bather has the hope that this therapy will ease the pain. But sharing a

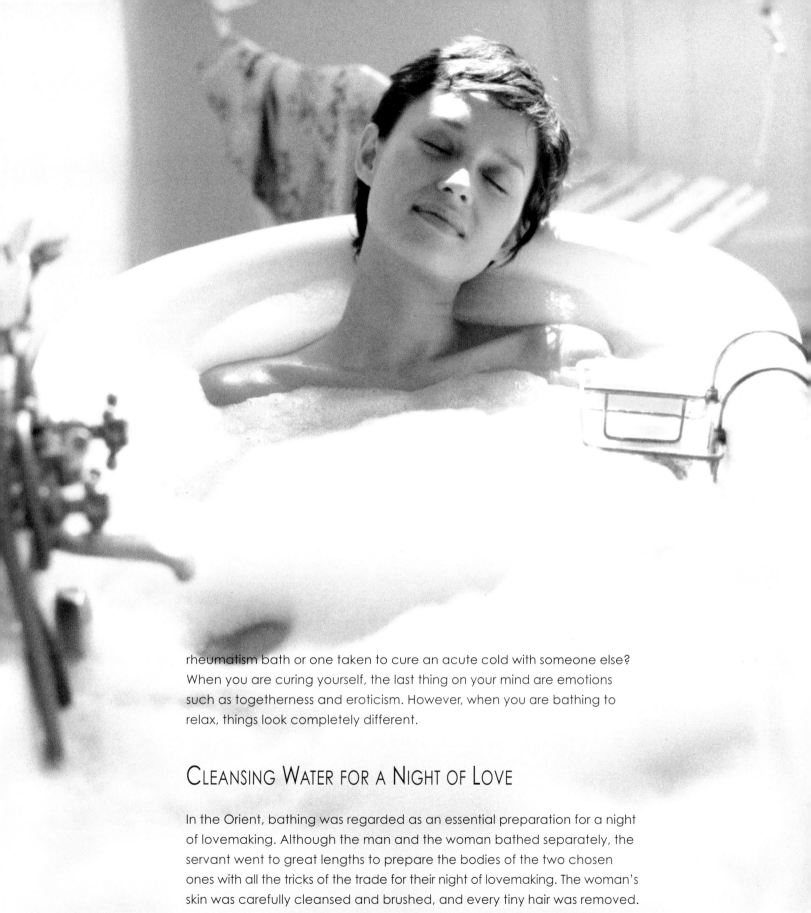

rheumatism bath or one taken to cure an acute cold with someone else? When you are curing yourself, the last thing on your mind are emotions such as togetherness and eroticism. However, when you are bathing to relax, things look completely different.

CLEANSING WATER FOR A NIGHT OF LOVE

In the Orient, bathing was regarded as an essential preparation for a night of lovemaking. Although the man and the woman bathed separately, the servant went to great lengths to prepare the bodies of the two chosen ones with all the tricks of the trade for their night of lovemaking. The woman's skin was carefully cleansed and brushed, and every tiny hair was removed.

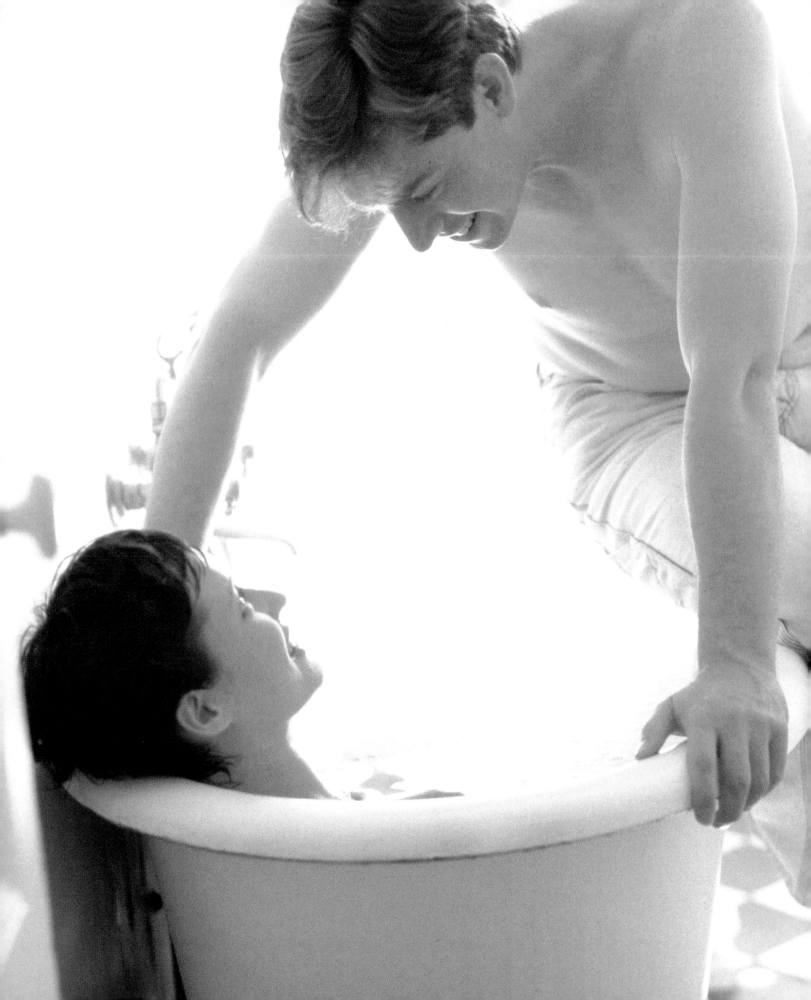

Then the servants rubbed the skin with henna to give it a lovely colour and make it silky smooth. Busy hands also prepared the man for his celebration of love. He wasn't treated quite as gently; instead he was rubbed all over with pumice to remove all flakes of dead skin. The man's skin was meant to feel as soft as silk to the woman's hands. The most important role in this fastidious cleansing ceremony was played by water, which envelops the naked body like an invisible cloak in a protective gesture and prevents it from shivering as it would in the open air.

A warm bath gives bathers the feeling that they have found their inner self, protected as they were so many years before in their mother's womb. But this feeling can of course be extended to two people who have a special relationship. They embrace and touch one another, trace the contours of the partner's body with their fingertips and kiss. Under the hot shower or together in the bath, a very special feeling of togetherness is generated between the two partners. It is said that food keeps body and soul together – when two people who love and yearn for one another bathe together, the water holds their bodies and souls together. There will be moments when they have the sensation of being one – one body and one soul.

There is a wide range of sensations that one can feel when bathing with a loved one. It can include just splashing around or a furious water battle with hilarious laughter or passionate massaging and stroking – ending in mutual meditation, in which both partners close their eyes and experience their partner's closeness.

Admittedly, the bubbling pleasure does not come on its own, neither does the almost mystical absorption or erotic passion. It is necessary to make some preparations and considerations as to the dramaturgy of a mutual bathing celebration – unless of course the partners are natural talents in the subject of bathing and lovemaking, or they have developed a routine in bathing together.

FLEEING FROM THE DAY-TO-DAY DRUDGERY

The time of day is a crucial factor to the success of the mutual bathing pleasure. It may be the case that two young people who have just fallen in love end up tearing each other's clothes off the very moment they enter the hotel room and chase each other under the shower to let their passions run wild without thinking too long or hard about the situation. However, leaving aside such dramatic moments as these, bathing together must be done at a time when one knows that one is not liable to be disturbed and when the schedules for the following day are banished from one's mind.

Passion is spontaneous and cannot be planned, but one can of course give some special care and attention to the place that is to offer the opportunity for a night of passion.

If your bath is just large enough for one person, it is of course pointless insisting on a bath together with your partner. On the other hand, that does not mean that you have to do without a fulfilled bathing experience. You could take a comfortable chair into the bathroom and first let your partner climb into the bath. The man can help the woman undress or just sit back and watch her lovingly as she undresses herself. This can be an exciting experience in itself.

The partners can simply talk to each other – after all, they have all the time in the world and the evening is young. They can exchange dreams or invent and compare fantasies. He can serve her, fetch her a refreshing drink, a tasty snack or some cool fruit. He can gently and lovingly massage her neck and back, wash her hair and let his fingertips wander idly over her scalp. And eventually she can return all these favours – and quite a few more besides.

It can be an absolutely wonderful experience to be pampered by some-one you love, just lying there with your eyes closed, fully trusting your partner. Both partners could also stand in the bath and dry each other off, catch drops of water with their lips – erotic games, childish games, but filled with tenderness.

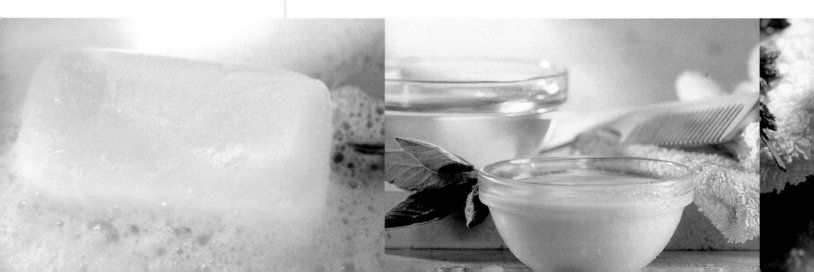

The Suitable Ambience for Your Private Bath Festivity

A bathing celebration for two people in love could be compared with an opera. This might seem a little exaggerated when you think of some of the bathrooms you have seen – small white-tiled enclosures that give you just enough space to stand beside the mirror and brush your teeth and for the occasional shower. But why not exaggerate for once, quite deliberately, and allow yourself the eccentric luxury of creating your very own bathing temple at home. The secret is that you don't have to plan a new bathroom that looks like it came straight out of a lifestyle magazine. That would be far too expensive and is not our intention. You can create your own personal temple to your own taste with a few small but effective ideas that all work together in harmony. The rest is up to your imagination. The budget really does not matter. A red rose in a champagne glass, a pink terry towel on the towel rack, a few drops of rose oil in the vaporiser: these are just three touches to stimulate your fantasy, the piers supporting the bridge of your imagination.

Every sense should be stimulated: what you see and hear, the aroma and the taste and also what you touch.

For this occasion you will need the appropriate setting; this is where you can really give your imagination free rein. Consider your bathroom as the recuperation centre of your apartment. Professional bathing institutions have long since discarded the purely functional interior design of the past and now provide fantastic landscapes with grottoes hidden away among palm trees, finnish saunas, waterfalls running over rocky landscapes...
You don't have to turn your bathroom into an elaborate landscape, but take up the general idea and stop thinking of your bathroom as merely a place for personal hygiene. It should be the refuge in your home – a place where you can go to relax and recharge your batteries.

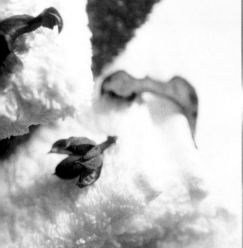
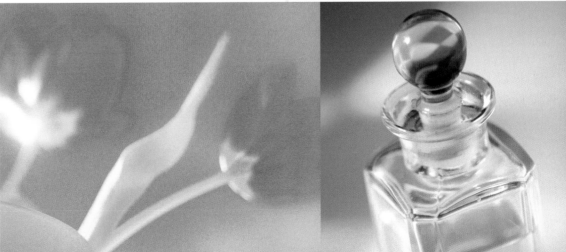

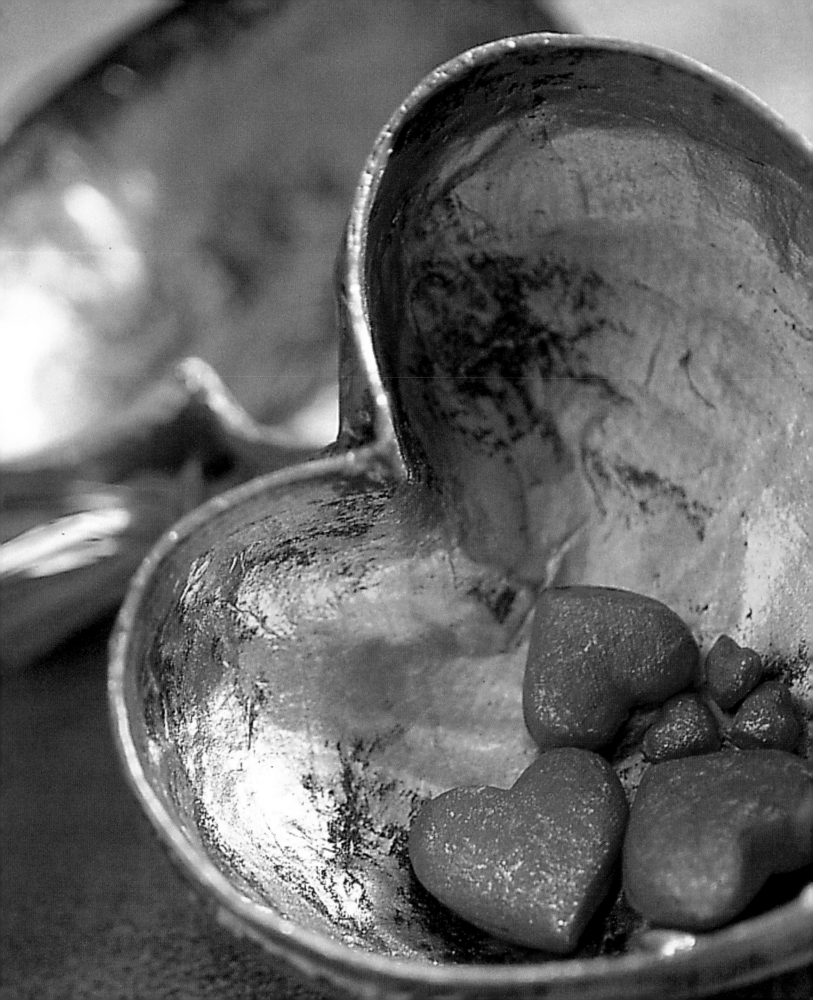

On the other hand, you will have to do something about this yourself; after all, a normal bathroom is not exactly predestined to allow two people to withdraw and forget all about the world around them. Of course, if you are the lucky owner of a modern, tastefully designed bathroom, things will be simpler for you. You only have to bother about the accessories that set the scene for love.

Think of flowers. If you have enough room, you could always have a plant standing in a suitable position in the bathroom. But even a bunch of flowers in a vase makes a colourful and perhaps aromatic statement. And for your love bath, you should select a very special flower arrangement, different from the flowers that normally decorate the room. As the saying goes, less can often be more: a single long-stemmed rose in a long narrow crystal vase or some rose petals in a bowl might be just what you both want. Bath oils, eau de toilette, essences, shampoos and lotions are usually sold in unsightly plastic bottles. Don't place these boring containers on the side of the bath or on the windowsill: buy some attractive carafes, bottles and bowls into which you can pour the ingredients. If you want to open your own aroma oil bar to create your very own cocktails, these bottles are every effective when placed together on a shelf. There are many different types, shapes and colours of soap, and bath oils in gelatine balls that can be kept in a bowl or an attractive storage glass. Wander through the glassware department of your local department store, and look for the most beautiful glass vessels for your bathing paradise.

Don't be afraid to buy accessories that would seem to be quite useless – if you like them, buy them. You do not have to justify your decision to anybody if you buy a silver comb at a flea market, glass dolphins or stone ladybirds. Apart from that, a variety of stones can produce a wonderful effect and emanate powers that you can feel, something you would never have believed possible before. How about a colourful mat on top of the tiles, an acrylic towel rack, a mussel-shaped soap dish – and by the way, why shouldn't the window have curtains, perhaps organza curtains that set a playful, colourful accent? Why not buy some sparkling coat hangers? An atomiser made of lava stone? An arabesque mirror? There are so many different possibilities – after all, the most beautiful things in life are those that you really like.

Different colours create different moods. Pastel tones make relatively small rooms seem more spacious, because they let the light flow in. Dimmed lamps or the light from flickering candles create a mysterious stillness and

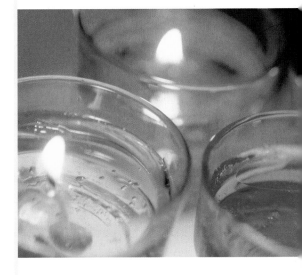

candlelight gives your body a bronze taint, making bare skin beautiful and seductive.

It is important that you create your own style; you must find pleasure in the atmosphere. You should simply feel good – this is why there are no generally applicable rules of the game. If you love vivid colours or extreme contrasts, then do not be afraid to say so. Your bath oasis is your very personal place, where no one will criticise or judge you.

Gentle Tones like the Rushing of a Stream

Of course, you will need some music for your bath festivity – but not just any old music from the radio, interrupted by annoying advertisements and announcements. Someone speaking in the background will distract you from the matter at hand, because even without wanting to, you will find yourself unconsciously listening to what is being said. And nothing is worse for the mutual bathing pleasure than when your intellect is addressed suddenly and you begin a lengthy discussion about what is being said on the radio. Sitting in the lovely warm water – two bodies close together – is an experience of the emotions. Your conscious thoughts must be switched off and be completely replaced by feelings.

It is often said that singing is a distracting factor. For any type of meditation the rule is that only instrumental music will allow you to reach a trance-like

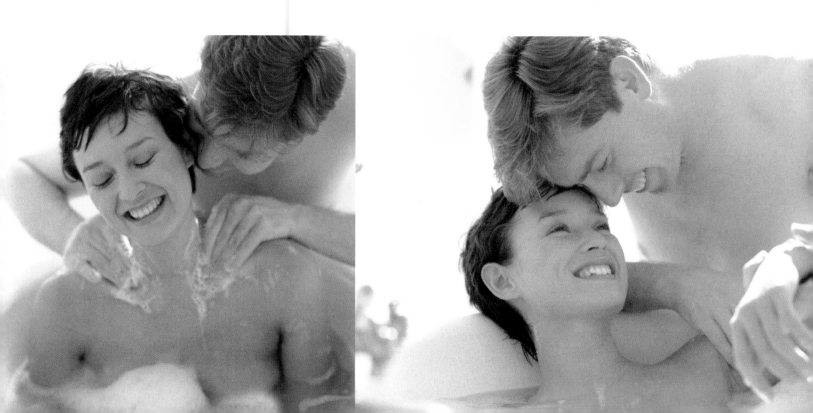

state, far removed from reality. On the other hand, this shouldn't be taken too seriously; it should rather depend on the needs of the bathers. A young couple may find top-ten hits suitable for their raucous water games, while others are entranced when they listen to an opera aria. And why shouldn't a couple like listening to bagpipe music in the bath? Everyone must decide for himself or herself – but of course the two partners have to agree. If only one partner enjoys the musical background, it will be difficult for both to concentrate on one another.

You can bring many different sounds into your bath world with a small CD player. However, if you are looking for a musical background that does not completely take over the bathing experience but merely stimulates the feelings of both partners in an unassuming manner and helps them to turn their backs on the outside world and concentrate on their own inner feelings, meditation music is highly recommended. Music stores and even some bookshops and esoteric shops have a large selection of this type of music with relaxing sounds. Particularly beautiful are compositions that introduce natural sounds – such as the sounds of morning beside a lake with birds singing and the whisper of the water – into a small bathroom, thus transforming the loving couple's environment into a magical wonder-land. If you close your eyes and sit back and relax inwardly as well as out-wardly, feel the water on your body and the physical closeness of your partner, this is a wonderful framework for absolute relaxation, to rediscover the closeness of your loved one and recharge your batteries far away from the drudgery of everyday life. Usually this music is played quietly, as

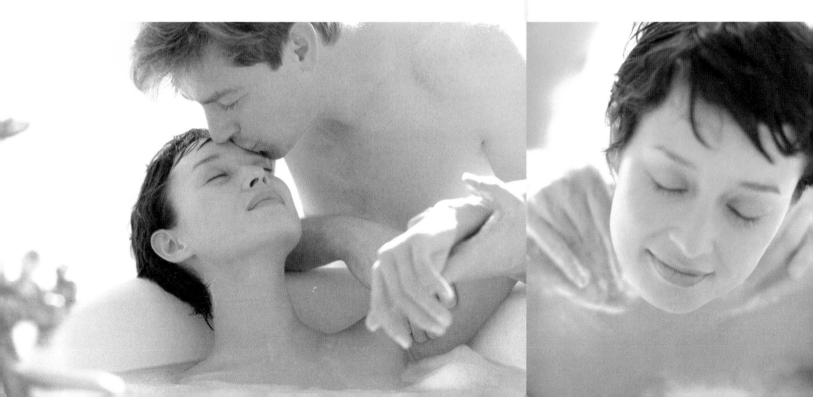

an almost imperceptible background accompaniment. Nothing would ruin the sensuous moment more than if you were literally overwhelmed by the music.

Talking is permitted. Probably you both want to talk about how your day has been; perhaps one of you has had a silly, amusing experience. It is better if you agree not to discuss anything too serious. Some couples end up arguing very quickly if they have opposing opinions on a specific matter. You know each other – avoid talking about or doing anything that could spoil the mood. Problems can wait until another time. After all, you want to strengthen one another so that you can master all problems with renewed energy.

Compliment each other. Tell your partner just what it is that you find so wonderful about him or her, how much you love and admire him or her. Express your feelings. This is a good topic for bathing together: bring your feelings to the surface and simply allow your partner to be part of them. Talk about yourself and your partner. Remember the most beautiful moments of your time together. List everything that you have in common. Talk about how and when you first met and when you realised that you were in love, what your partner means to you. You could also take this opportunity to apologise for an unnecessary argument, for ignoring your partner's wishes, or for your own bad habits. Talk about your relationship, how wonderful it is and how it could be even better. But leave your problems outside the bathroom door.

Perhaps this little bath celebration will bring you closer to each other again. You have been ignoring one another for some time or perhaps you have had an argument, but now you have both decided to throw everything that has been causing the problems out of the bathroom. Naked as you both are, open up your souls to one another and really make up.

But it can also be good when you both just sit there without talking, communicating solely with smiles and gestures. You will probably find that you talk more with each other at the start of your bath celebration and that the words will slowly dry up as you pamper each other with bath essences and gentle touching.

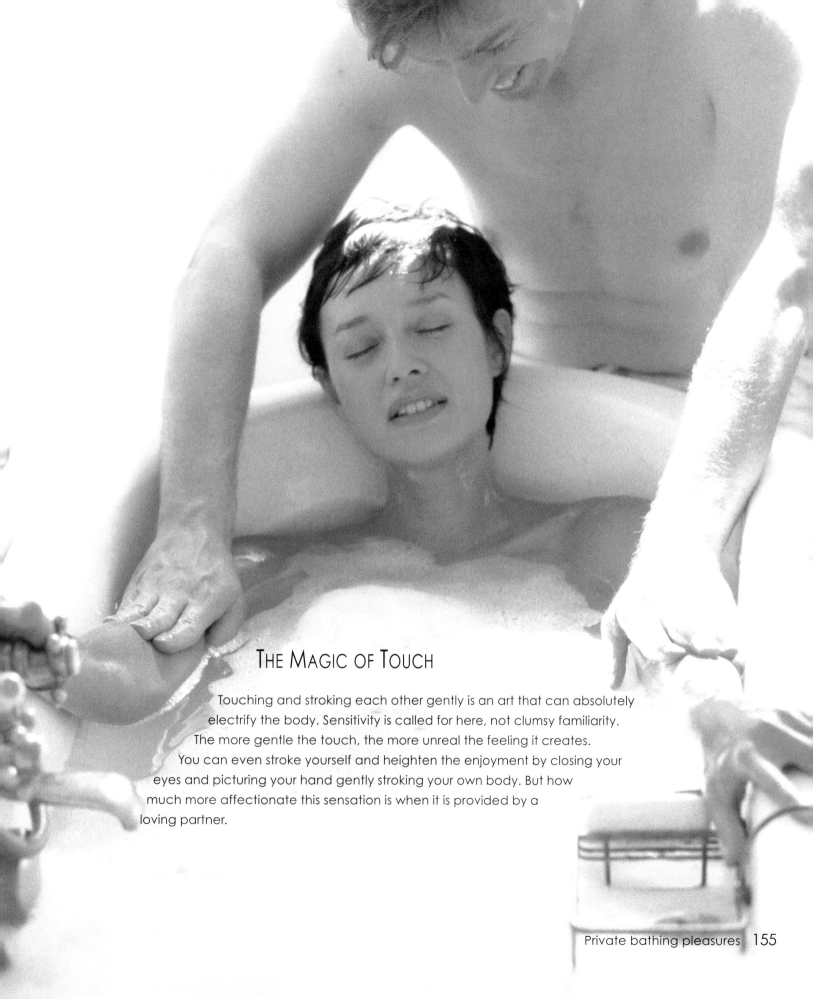

THE MAGIC OF TOUCH

Touching and stroking each other gently is an art that can absolutely
electrify the body. Sensitivity is called for here, not clumsy familiarity.
The more gentle the touch, the more unreal the feeling it creates.
You can even stroke yourself and heighten the enjoyment by closing your
eyes and picturing your hand gently stroking your own body. But how
much more affectionate this sensation is when it is provided by a
loving partner.

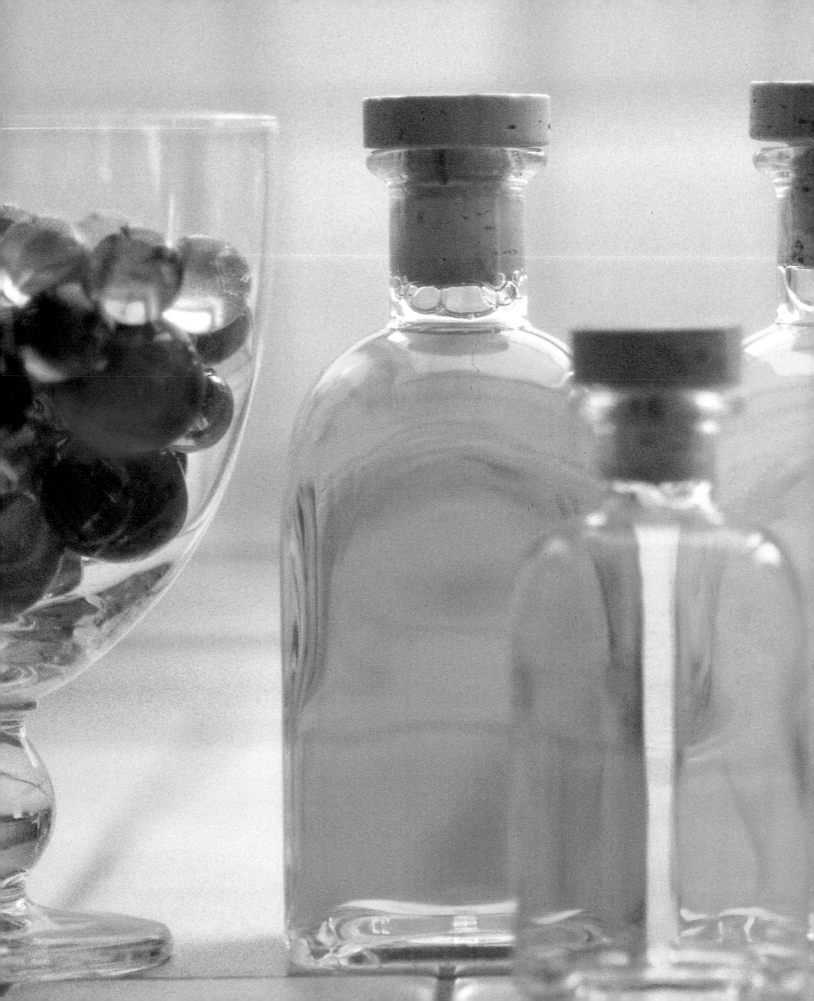

You and your partner can massage each other while you are in the bath or when drying yourselves off afterwards – no matter whether you are standing, sitting or lying down. She can sit on the edge of the tub or on a stool. He then stands behind her and massages her back, shoulders and neck. Or both stand facing each other massaging each other's back. Once your skin is dry you can rub in a lovely fragrant massage oil. It is much more pleasant than massaging dry skin. And besides this, your skin needs to replace some oil.

No one expects you to be as good as a professional masseur. Of course, it is sensible to make yourselves familiar with the most important massage techniques and can distinguish between stroking, kneading and pressing. But in this very special situation you will find that you massage quite in-tuitively. You will immediately know if your partner is enjoying your touch or if it is uncomfortable. If you massage one another at the same time, you will find that you automatically synchronise your massaging movements and fall into a rhythm. You are sure to massage each other with a lot of feeling – after all, each touch is an expression of the tenderness and love that you feel for one another.

Aromas to Bewitch the Soul

The majority of bath essences have a very intensive aroma, particularly when they are made from essential oils. Nevertheless, these aromatic oils can be used to create a very pleasant atmosphere in the room. In order to create aromas such as these, you will need a vaporiser. This is nothing more than a ceramic bowl with a candle or tea light below, or sometimes it is an electric heating plate which keeps the water warm. You then add a few drops of the essential oils of your choice to the water bowl. As the oil dissolved in the water evaporates, this creates the distinctive aroma that fills the room. Normally a mixture of different oils is used, depending on just what type of aroma you want to create and the effect you intend to achieve.

Of course, you could also place spices in the warm water of the vaporiser – for instance juniper berries, cloves, caraway, aniseed, vanilla pods, car-damom pods, coriander, nutmeg, ginger root, lemon, orange or lime peel, star aniseed or allspice. Whether the aroma is to be pure or mixed with other aromas is a matter for the individual to decide. There are simply no limits to creativity.

Of course, you should refrain from burning cerain substances, such as herbs or woods, if you are allergic to them.

Another method of creating pleasant aromas is by burning some incense or other substances. This is one of the oldest customs known to man and is still practised today in a number of different cultures, for instance in Arabia and Egypt, by native Americans, and of course in China and Japan, in India and Tibet. In all of these countries, certain methods of burning these substances have developed in thousand-year-old traditions. However, they all have one thing in common: precious woods, resins and herbs are burned to create the desired scent. There are many different reasons for using incense. It can be used to disinfect the room, purify the air or to alleviate physical and mental problems. Incense is also used to create a meditative atmosphere, of course also to intensify the contact between individual people and between humans and nature.

In India, people have always valued the stimulating power of aromas while succumbing to the effects of an erotic massage. To heighten your passion, use mixtures of aloe, cardamom, cloves, sandalwood, patchouli, benjamin gum and frankincense. In the Himalayan region, people traditionally use galgangal, ginger, mugwort, dwarf juniper and thistles.

Many substances have a very intensive aroma and are thus less suitable for the bathing ceremony. But everyone must decide for themselves which aromas they especially like or dislike. Because of the nature of water, the aromatic magic of essential oils may be more harmonious than an aroma that is created by burning a fragrant substance. Incense is perhaps more suited to meditative situations than to enhancing the atmosphere of a mutual lovemaking bath.

Beneficial aromas can also be created without evaporation or combustion, by spreading certain spices and dried herbs in bowls or sewing them into textiles – usually cushions. The type of mixture depends on the desired aroma. For a fresh and spicy mood, you could make up a potpourri of bay leaf, basil, mint, juniper berries, star aniseed and lemon and orange peel. Just remember not to overdo it.

In the dining room, an intensive aroma is not so desirable, because your appetite will quickly be spoiled if the aroma and taste of the food are overlaid with the scent of the potpourri.

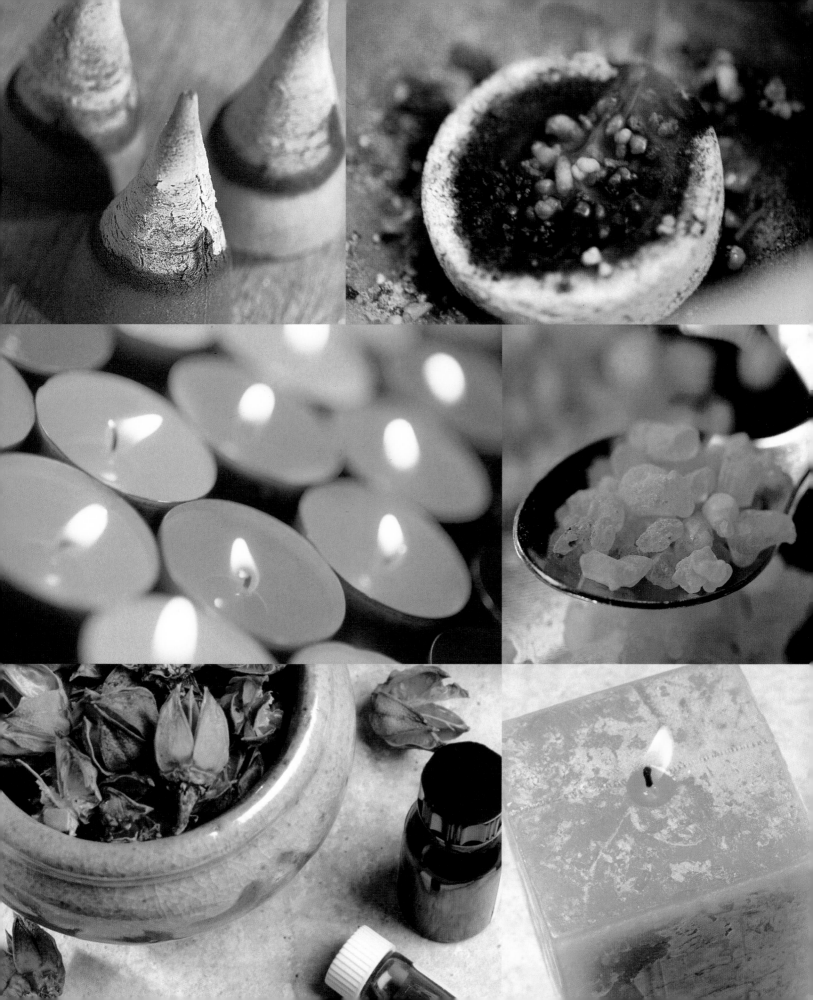

Essence of Love

3 tablespoons of olive oil
5 drops of muscatel sage oil
1 drops of black pepper
4 drops of jasmine oil

A bath for a cold winter's day, when the landscape is covered in snow, icicles are hanging from the roof and the sky is a milky-grey colour. In a jam jar, mix the olive oil with two very different essential oils – five drops of muscatel sage oil with its sweet, fresh aroma and one drop of oil from black pepper with its fiery, exciting scent. Four drops of jasmine oil reduce the contrast and melt the duo of oils into a magical essence of love.

Baths for Two

An Exotic Rose Bath

5 drops of muscatel sage oil
3 drops of ylang-ylang oil
3 drops of rose oil

Essential oils of rose, muscatel sage and ylang-ylang are mixed in olive oil. The exotic ylang-ylang oil dominates this mixture with its distinct fragrance, while the gentle scent of rose floats just above it in the background. This bath encourages shy people and gives them the opportunity of throwing fears and despondency overboard and fulfilling their most secret dreams.

Bubbling Bath of Love

3 drops of lemon oil
3 drops of rose oil
5 drops of cardamom oil
10 g ($^1/_3$ oz) soda
10 g ($^1/_3$ oz) sodium bicarbonate
5 g ($^1/_6$ oz) sodium perborate

This scent consists of three drops of rose oil, five drops of cardamom oil and three drops of lemon oil. Cardamom is the driving force of these three ingredients – it is reputed to be one of the most effective aphrodisiacs. If you add 10 g ($^1/_3$ oz) of soda, 10 g ($^1/_3$ oz) of sodium bicarbonate and 5 g ($^1/_6$ oz) of sodium perborate and mix everything into the bath water, it does not just smell seductive – the addition of sodium perborate starts a chemical reaction with the oxygen contained in the bath water, and the water begins to bubble. There is a tingling sensation on the skin of the two lovers, which is transformed into an expression of their tension and expectations.

BATH FOR PASSION

Take four or five pieces of cinnamon bark and prepare an infusion with boiling water. Pour this through a sieve into a porcelain container and add three drops of balm oil, three drops of lemon oil and three drops of sandalwood oil. This mixture is then poured into the bath. Scatter a handful of balm leaves on the surface of the water. Cinnamon, an Indian ingredient for love, dominates this mixture and intensifies the two bathers' desire for each other.

4–5 pieces of cinnamon bark
3 drops of balm oil
3 drops of lemon oil
3 drops of sandalwood oil
Balm leaves (dried)

HONEY LAVENDER BATH

Combine one cup of honey with four drops of ylang-ylang, two drops of lavender and two drops of sandalwood. Mix the ingredients well. If you like, you can also scatter a handful of dried lavender into the bath water. This bath is ideal for overly excited lovers since this mixture has a pleasantly calming effect.

1 cup of honey
4 drops of ylang-ylang oil
2 drops of lavender oil
2 drops of sandalwood oil

SENSUAL BATH

Mix three drops of ylang-ylang with 10 g ($^1/_3$ oz) of grapeseed oil. Add one drop of pure rose oil and two drops of pure grapefruit oil. The ylang-ylang tree, which grows to a height of 25 metres (about 70 feet), has strongly smelling flowers that are said to have a powerful effect as an aphrodisiac. This oil with its antiseptic effect also calms the digestive tract during infections and supports the regeneration of the nervous system.

3 drops of ylang-ylang
10 ml ($^1/_3$ oz) grapeseed oil
1 drop of rose oil
2 drops of grapefruit oil

SANDALWOOD BATH

The warm and velvety fragrance of sandalwood oil transports us into tropical forests and oriental palaces. Sandalwood has deep, soft vibrations and a balancing and harmonising effect, especially during times of emotional stress. The signals of its fragrance are unsurpassed in encouraging personal contact. When filling the bath, add the milk powder and honey to the stream of water. As soon as the bath is filled, mix sandalwood oil and rose oil into the water. Sandalwood oil – mixed with a neutral oil – is also very well suited for a massage.

6 tablespoons of goat's milk
(preferably in powder form)
2 tablespoons of honey
3 drops of sandalwood oil
3 drops of rose oil

A Culinary Climax

The old adage that one should never go bathing on a full stomach also applies to the bath of passion. However, you do not have to go to bed with an empty stomach after your watery pleasures are over – on the contrary: what you did without before can now be enjoyed twice as much as you are now physically and mentally recharged. The sensuous bath is followed by an exciting dinner that really gets passions high and nourishes the fire of love.

Of course, if you feel like it you can have a snack while you are bathing. Because you cannot remain in the water for longer than twenty minutes without getting wrinkly skin, you will not have time for any great banquets along with the bathing ritual. At the most, you can enjoy a cracker with caviar or some fruit, but you can also nibble on some pieces of red or green pepper, celery or asparagus. However, no one would really enjoy indulging in a large feast in the bathwater.

However, after your bath you should not just run into the kitchen and appease your hunger by quickly grabbing some butter, cheese and cold cuts from the fridge and sitting or standing at the bench eating a few sandwiches. Like the bath, everything should be staged carefully – after all, you have to arrange the next act.

Not everything that you normally like is suitable for such a meal. Robust plain-fare cooking such as roast beef with roast potatoes and yorkshire pudding would hardly be a fitting end to your fantastic passionate festivities. If you fill your stomach with such ballast, your organism will be fully occupied with digesting this culinary impertinence. Then you and your partner will think of nothing else but dropping into bed exhausted and falling asleep immediately. The food must be light and well-devised in regard to combination, taste and presentation. Presentation is very important: you really should come up with something really special. It doesn't have to be caviar – even simple ingredients, presented in an interesting way, can create a similar passion in the dining room to the ardour you have already experienced in the aromatic bath water.

Through their shape, colour and aroma alone, exotic fruits express sensuous joy. Think of papayas, passionfruit or figs. There is a good reason why the fig is regarded as a symbol of fertility in Mediterranean countries. Pick up a fig, cut

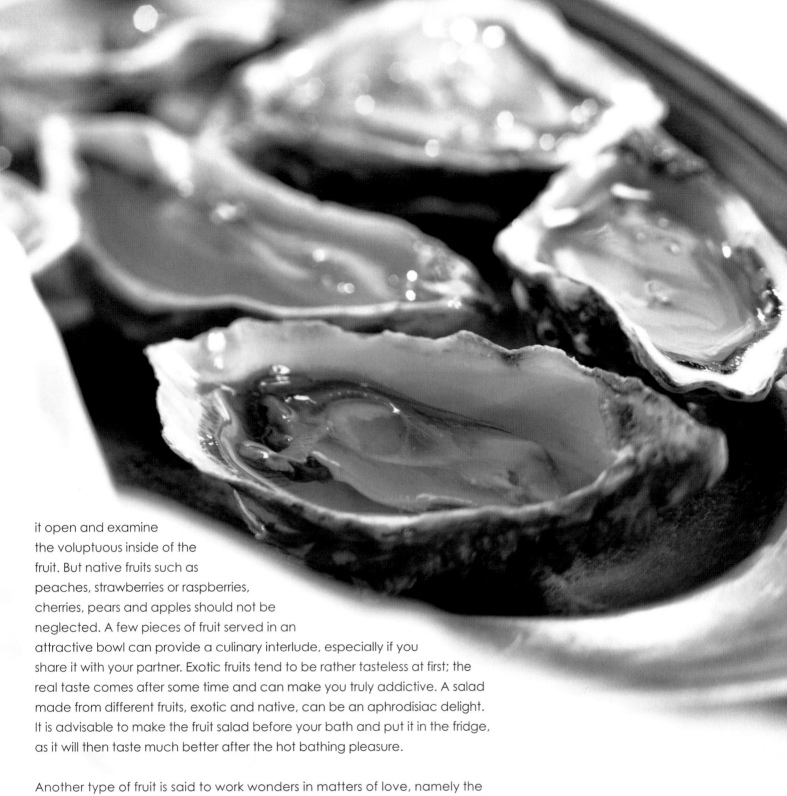

it open and examine
the voluptuous inside of the
fruit. But native fruits such as
peaches, strawberries or raspberries,
cherries, pears and apples should not be
neglected. A few pieces of fruit served in an
attractive bowl can provide a culinary interlude, especially if you
share it with your partner. Exotic fruits tend to be rather tasteless at first; the
real taste comes after some time and can make you truly addictive. A salad
made from different fruits, exotic and native, can be an aphrodisiac delight.
It is advisable to make the fruit salad before your bath and put it in the fridge,
as it will then taste much better after the hot bathing pleasure.

Another type of fruit is said to work wonders in matters of love, namely the
fruits of the sea. Seafood does in fact contain vast amounts of protein. It is
said that Casanova ate three dozen oysters a day to keep his testosterone
level high. Besides protein, oysters also contain plenty of zinc, while mussels
contain iron and iodine. Moreover, it is undeniably a sensuous pleasure to
enjoy the tasty shellfish in their hard shells.

One should not be too miserly when preparing the dinner for two; caviar is also an ideal accompaniment. The table does not have to be overflowing with delicacies. It is not the quantity that is important; the subtle details are really what make the difference.

SECRETS OF EROTIC CUISINE

A little luxury never hurts and it is important for the soul, especially when you are spending an unforgettable evening together. Buy a truffle. Just the thought of having spent money on such a luxury is already something special; in addition, these tubers contain psychoactive substances with a chemical structure similar to that of pheromones, the human sexual lures.

Vegetables can look enticing and as far as their effects as aphrodisiacs are concerned, many other foodstuffs cannot hold a candle to them. Asparagus is a good example. Its main constituent, asparagine, has a diuretic effect and also heightens passion. Besides this, asparagus is an exceptionally light vegetable. Celery contains potassium, sodium and phosphorus, all minerals that really get the love carousel into its rhythm. There is also the strange bitter taste. The sexual lure eberpheromone, which is present in celeriac, has a libido-stimulating effect. The bitter substance cynarine contained in artichokes also gives it its stimulating taste. One of the most important effects of the artichoke is its stimulating effect on the blood circulation throughout the whole body, making you fit for your night of passion.

Finally you must consider using the right herbs and spices for your dinner: dill, for example, or parsley, basil and rosemary. Everyone is familiar with these common kitchen herbs, but few people know that they do not just have a characteristic taste and smell but that the substances present in the herbs chase away listlessness and arouse your appetite for love. The reason for this is that they contain bitter substances and tannin as well as essential oils, all in tiny but effective doses. The spices in the rack spice up your love life not just because they have a hot taste, but because their biochemical constituents noticeably increase your sensitivity to erotic stimulation. Pepper contains piperine, chilli has capsaicine and ginger contains gingerol. Dishes made with these hot oriental spices send your blood hurtling through your veins and activate your metabolism. Even the normally most calm and collected person will soon have fire surging through his or her body. Or add a pinch of nutmeg to a cup of hot milk or cardamom in hot coffee – these two remedies are guaranteed to heighten your passion.

And of course, the presentation makes a big difference. As decoration, place a nicely shaped red chilli pepper on the plate, even if you don't dare bite into this hot vegetable. Shapes and colours stimulate our subconscious desire for love. When a woman runs her fingers over an avocado or slowly slides a fig into her mouth she is sending out a clear signal that should get any hot-blooded male going.

ROOM FOR LOVE

It doesn't really matter where you retire to after the bath. The main thing is that you should feel comfortable there. On a balmy summer evening, nothing is nicer than relaxing on the balcony or the patio, or perhaps you have a gazebo at the bottom of the garden. Maybe your favourite place is a cosy corner in the living room. Or perhaps you feel like building yourself a cave from cushions and sitting on the floor with a white tablecloth spread out between you. Have a picnic in the lounge. Forget the dining table, just make yourself cosy.

Of course no one is stopping you setting the table to celebrate the occasion with your most expensive damask tablecloth, your best set of porcelain plates, crystal glasses and silver cutlery.

But then again it doesn't have to be a carefully laid-out table. You can just as easily lay out plates, glasses, cutlery and the food on a small coffee table or spread it out on the floor. The only important thing is that it is done with loving care.

Another idea is that instead of placing a vase of flowers on the table you could decorate it with a bunch of fresh herbs. Parsley, coriander, basil, mint, lemon balm is an aromatic potpourri that frees the head and opens up the soul. Or you could simply let some flower petals swim around in a bowl of water, perhaps together with some floating candles. Roses are not just lovely to look at when arranged in a vase; rose petals scattered over the table are also a highly effective form of decoration.

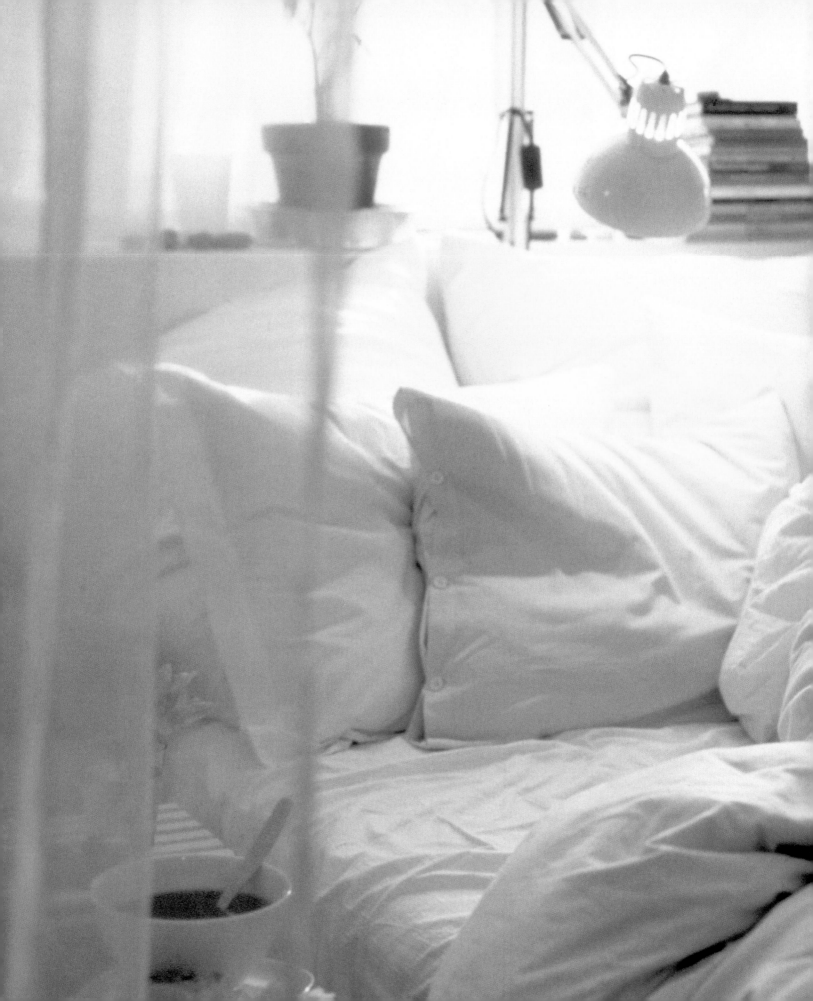

You could also prepare some digestive spices in a glass bowl. Mix aniseed, fennel, coriander and caraway seeds and roast them in a pot. You can nibble at these seeds during the meal. This aids digestion, makes you feel good and freshens your breath.

You can leave the lights on if you are able to dim them. A standing lamp that only radiates a dull glow is also quite suitable. Of course, you can simply enjoy the warm glow of several candles. Electric light spoils the atmosphere. When your partner is veiled in a cloak of darkness, he or she takes on a mysterious image which increases your desire for each other. Go along with this game. Keep your distance. Enjoy the feeling of expectation, extend the pleasure. The longer you celebrate the banquet of passion, the better the climax. You are feeling good and you should enjoy this feeling as long as possible.

Love needs space, so that your feelings for your partner have room to unfold. Passion that gradually develops is more substantial than spontaneous gratificaction. Of course, when you are ravenous, you simply jam everything into your mouth and are full within a few minutes. However, a gourmet meal requires time, and every minute, every hour increases the passion until it becomes almost unbearable. If you take your time dining, you are doing your body a favour. You will eat less and chew your food more thoroughly – in this way you will discover the true taste of the food you are eating.

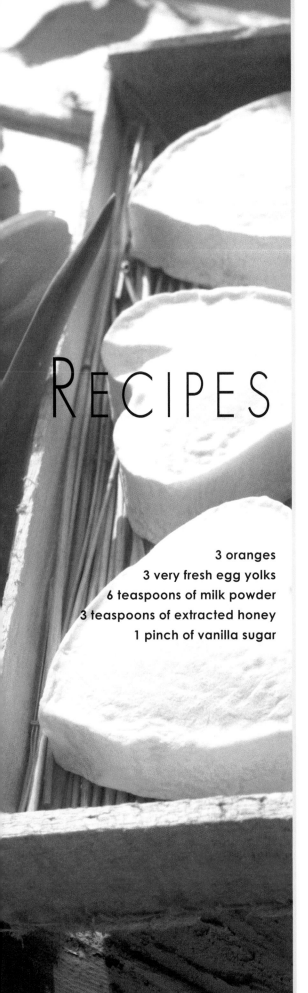

Cuisine d'Amour

There is of course some truth in the popular belief that it is possible to awaken passion in a person or even animate them to make love by feeding him or her certain foods. There must be a certain disposition beforehand, that tingling sensation – if this already exists, of course specific foods can work wonders and turn human nature haywire. To put it succinctly, "a good meal, a glass of wine, a passionate woman – that is the best way to spend an evening." This saying from an old tapestry expresses everything that makes up a wonderful evening of passion, a bath together and a sumptuous meal afterwards.

Recipes for Love

Entrée

3 oranges
3 very fresh egg yolks
6 teaspoons of milk powder
3 teaspoons of extracted honey
1 pinch of vanilla sugar

Squeeze the oranges and pour the juice along with the other ingredients (egg yolk, milk powder, honey and vanilla sugar) into the mixer. Mix the ingredients briefly.

Put split ice cubes into an elegant glass. Pour the frothy cocktail over the ice. Drink this alcohol-free drink with a red straw.

Tomato Soup with Black Olives

This delicious soup will stimulate you even further after a hot steaming bath and make you simply lust for love. First, the tomatoes need to be skinned. Then pour boiling water over them, briefly rinse them with cold water, and the skin can then be peeled off easily. Cut the tomatoes into cubes.

Peel the shallots and cut them into fine rings. Cook them in three tablespoonfuls of olive oil until they are transparent.

Now add the tomato cubes to the pot, cook for another two minutes and then add $1^{1}/_{2}$ pints of water. Cook over a low heat for half an hour. Finally, puree the soup with a hand-held electric mixer and pass it through a sieve. Season with pepper, salt and paprika powder to taste or round off with two tablespoonfuls of cream or crème fraîche. Stone the olives and briefly heat them in a frying pan with some olive oil. Pour the soup into soup bowls, distribute the olives evenly and garnish with a spoonful of crème fraîche.

1 kg (2 lb) tomatoes
2 bunches of shallots
4 tablespoons of olive oil
$^{3}/_{4}$ l ($1^{1}/_{2}$ pints) water
Salt, pepper, paprika powder
Crème fraîche
Pouring cream
1 jar of black olives

CELERIAC SOUP

Cut celeriac into thin slices and blanche in boiling water with sea salt and a little oil for five minutes. Put a thick garlic clove through the garlic press, add it to the warm butter and cook briefly, making sure that the garlic does not turn brown. Add the celeriac, dust with a little carob flower, stir and add consommé double. Cook over a low heat for approximately eight minutes. Whip in two egg yolks with crème fraîche and two pinches of mace, salt and pepper. Remove from the heat and stir in the vegetables. Serve in pre-warmed decorative soup bowls adorned with some red peppercorns and plenty of tender chervil leaves.

The same soup can be prepared as an aphrodisiac with tender fennel. Instead of chervil, use the finely chopped tender green of the fennel and add some lightly roasted walnuts.

2 small, young celeriacs
1 thick garlic clove
A little carob flour
2 large cups of consommé double
2 egg yolks
$^{1}/_{8}$ l ($^{1}/_{4}$ pint) crème fraîche
2 pinches of mace
2 tablespoons of butter or margarine
Salt, pepper
Red peppercorns
Chervil leaves

ARTICHOKE SALAD WITH CELERY

First, cut the pre-cooked artichoke hearts and celery into slices. Cook the celery slices and the asparagus tips slowly in olive oil and arrange together with truffle slices and artichoke hearts on plates. Mix crème fraîche, balsamic vinegar, oil, salt and pepper for the dressing and pour three-quarters of it over the salad.

Place the scampi around the salad on the edge of the plate. Put into the fridge and pour dressing over the salad again before serving.

2 artichoke hearts (pre-cooked)
1 celery stalk
Green asparagus tips (about 15)
Truffle slices
Crème fraîche
Balsamic vinegar
Olive oil, salt, pepper
4 scampi

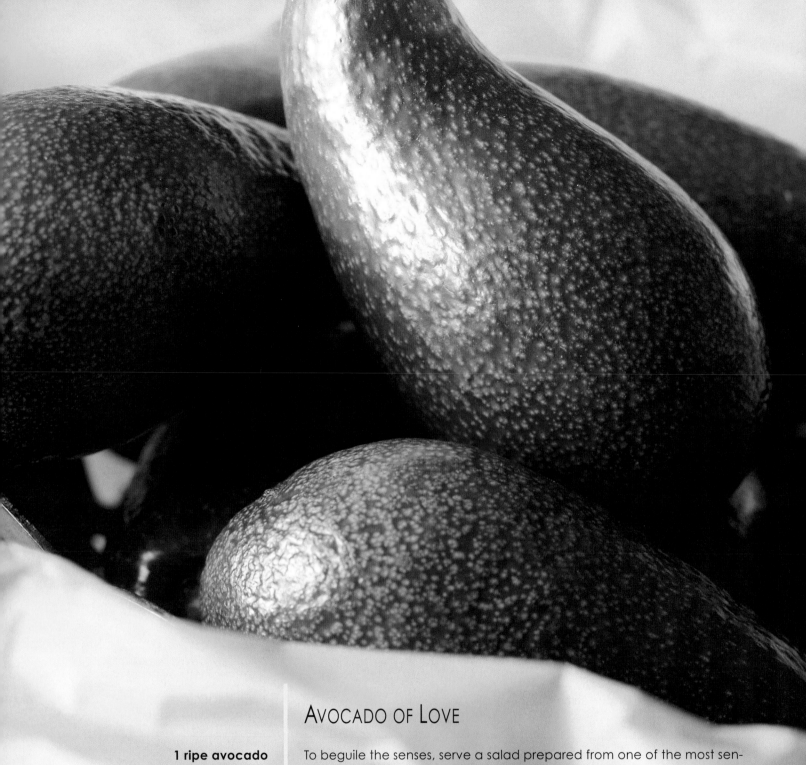

Avocado of Love

1 ripe avocado
1 tablespoon of colza oil
Balsamic vinegar
Salt, orange pepper
Mace for the vinaigrette
Juicy shrimps or sliced scampi

To beguile the senses, serve a salad prepared from one of the most sensual fruits of all – the avocado. Halve the ripe avocado lengthways with a sharp knife and discard the stone. With a small spoon, carefully remove the ripe flesh from the skin and cut it into tiny cubes. Fold in the vinaigrette prepared in advance, grind some nutmeg over the avocado and then decorate it with small shrimps and sliced scampi. Leave the salad to stand for approximately half an hour. Just before serving, pour some more vinaigrette over it.

Loup de Mer à la Casanova

Mix all ingredients with the olive oil and rub into the inside and outside of the fish. If you only have a fillet, let it marinate for at least two hours. If the fish is still in its skin, it must be cut in several places so that the marinade can soak in. Put the bouquet of savoury into the inside. Place the fish in a ceramic container, pour the mixture over it and cook in a hot oven for approximately 40 minutes. The fish can be served with coriander potatoes and lemon slices.

2 lb fresh loup de mer
1 bouquet of savoury
2 red onions
Olive oil
1 grated garlic clove
Thyme, bay leaf, sea salt
Orange pepper
Juice of 2 limes
1 pinch of cayenne pepper

Neptune's Fortune

Skin the john dory fillet carefully. Rub it with the garlic clove and cut the fish into thick cubes, which are then seasoned. Add them to a pre-heated frying pan that should not be too hot, and cook while constantly stirring. Add the white wine and then saffron and crème fraîche. Cook on low heat for five minutes and garnish with dill.

This dish goes well with fine mushrooms, such as fresh black truffle slices or morels cut into rings and cooked in butter, or a cep or oyster mushroom salad with garlic and continental parsley prepared in advance.

700 g (1$^1/_2$ lb) john dory fillet
1 garlic clove
Salt, pepper
Butter or margarine
White wine
Saffron
Crème fraîche
Dill

Chicken Liver for Lovers

Clean the chicken livers, let them dry on kitchen roll and lightly fry in olive oil with thyme, savoury, oregano, lovage and coriander. It is important to use either fresh herbs or herbs marinated in oil. Use at least three of the five herbs mentioned. Add some rich red wine. The dish should cook briefly over a medium heat before stirring in the crème fraîche. Remove the pot from the heat and then add sea salt and orange pepper.

Garnish with fresh basil – this makes for a tasty accent and is a pleasure for the eye. Serve the liver on warm wholemeal bread.

500 g (1 lb) chicken livers
Olive oil
Thyme, savoury, oregano,
lovage, coriander
A little red wine
Crème fraîche
Sea salt, orange pepper

Guinea Fowl Breast

4 guinea fowl breasts, unskinned
or 2 chicken breasts, skinned
Olive oil
Salt, orange pepper
Curry powder, cloves
Mace (ground)
1 tablespoon of balsamic vinegar
5 tablespoons of madeira
2 tablespoons of honey
Pouring cream
2 papayas or mangoes

Brown the pieces of guinea fowl breast on the skin side and season with sea salt, orange pepper, curry powder, cloves and nutmeg. After about four minutes turn over to the other side. If you use pieces of chicken breast, cut them into thick slices, season them and cook, making sure to turn them several times.

When the meat is cooked, add a mixture of aged balsamic vinegar, madeira and honey. Cook for approximately three minutes over a low heat. Finally add some pouring cream.

Serve with strips of papaya or mango that have been briefly cooked in butter. When served with fresh french stick, these breasts are a tender and stimulating dish.

Omlette Vitalité

3 large tomatoes
2 shallots
6 eggs
3 tablespoons of pouring cream
Olive oil or butter
1$^1/_2$ oz parmesan cheese

Skin the tomatoes, remove the seeds and cut into cubes. Cook the tomato cubes together with the chopped shallots in olive oil or butter. Remove the pot from the heat. Whisk cream and egg and add together with the tomatoes to a moderately heated frying pan. Stir the parmesan cheese and plenty of herbs (coriander, chervil, lemon balm, pimpernel, continental parsley and oregano) into the thickening eggs. You should use at

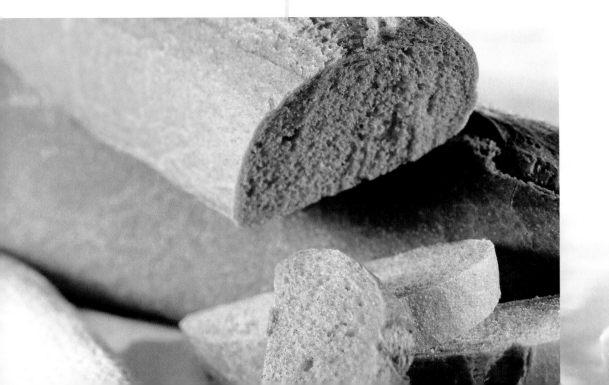

least three kinds of the herbs suggested. Finally season with sea salt and orange pepper.

The omelette must then be served immediately. Serve with fresh french stick bread.

Coriander, chervil, lemon balm, pimpernel, continental parsley, oregano
Sea salt, orange pepper

LOVE SNACKS

Prepare a few miniature sandwiches as snacks for the bath. As a basis, use toasted white bread cut into small triangles. These snacks should ideally be bite-sized. If you prefer, you could use round crackers instead of bread.

Spread the bread or crackers thinly with butter or margarine and then put some avocado puree and smoked salmon strips on a few of them. For the puree, mash two peeled avocados with a fork. Add plenty of lemon juice, to prevent the avocado flesh from turning brown. Season with freshly ground pepper.

Toast or crackers
Butter or margarine
1–2 avocados
2 oz smoked salmon
2 lemons
1 small tin of caviar
1 small onion
50 g (2 oz) smoked cheese
Dates

Decorate some more pieces of bread or crackers with caviar and a little onion ring. Drizzle with a little lemon juice. Put a slice of smoked cheese and a date (cut in half) on each of the remaining pieces. Everything should be nicely arranged on a tray and placed on a stool next to the bath tub.

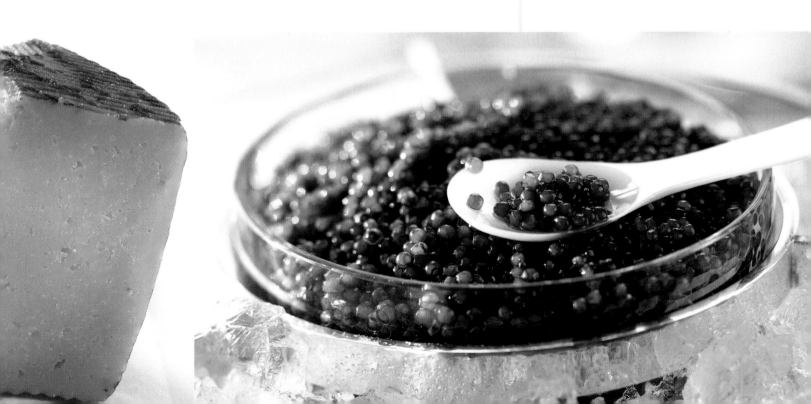

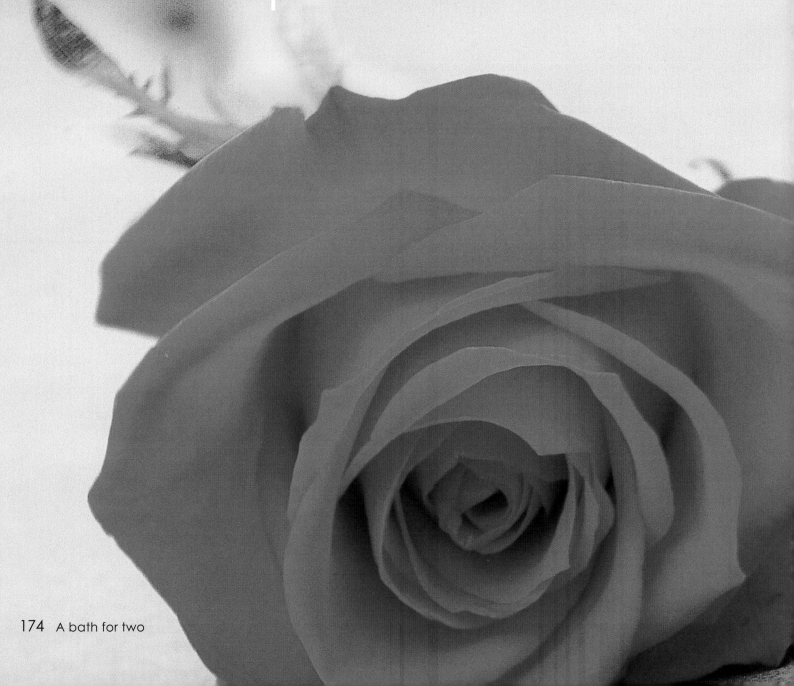

Rose Sorbet – a Sparkling Pleasure

**Juice and pulp of
a small lime or lemon
$^1/_8$ l ($^1/_2$ cup) refined sugar
10 ml ($^1/_3$ fl oz) raspberry brandy
2 drops of genuine rose oil
$^1/_4$ l ($^1/_2$ pint) champagne
1 egg white
Marrow of half a vanilla pod
1 fine rose**

The pulp and juice of a well-squeezed lime or half a lemon is mixed with half a cup of refined sugar. Let the sugar and juice come to the boil over a medium heat and put the mixture through a sieve. While the mixture is cooling, combine a glass of raspberry brandy with two drops of genuine rose oil. Pour this mixture into the syrup. The mixture is then filled into a sorbetière. Then carefully add the champagne and let this delicious mixture freeze slightly. Finally whip the egg white, add the marrow of a vanilla pod and carefully fold the beaten egg white into the sorbet. Put in the fridge for another five minutes.

The champagne glasses should be well chilled in the fridge. Before serving, put the petal of a fine rose into each glass. Then put the sorbet with a special ice-cream server or a deep tablespoon from the sorbetière into the champagne glasses. It is advisable to dip the ice-cream spoon briefly into hot water. Arrange the remaining rose petals elegantly on the saucers of the champagne glasses.

Apple Dream

Peel the apples and cut into small pieces. Cook in a pot with 100 ml ($3^1/_2$ fl oz) of water so that they become soft. Mash with a hand-held mixer or a fork. To make things easier for yourself, you can buy some ready-made apple sauce. In a separate pot, stir the fructose or honey into 250 ml ($^1/_2$ pint) of boiling water, then add the thyme leaves and let the mixture cook for five to ten minutes over a low heat. You can pour a splash of vodka into the syrup. As soon as the apple sauce and the syrup are cold, they are mixed together. Put the mixture into the freezer, but stir every half hour so that it remains nice and creamy and does not freeze to a solid block.

After four to five hours you can fill this delicious apple mixture with its un-rivalled thyme flavour into decorative glasses. If there is enough space in your fridge, put the glasses in there. With this drink, you can literally cool down after a hot bath which has heated up your body.

3–4 dessert apples
50 g (2 oz) fructose or honey
Fresh twigs of thyme
Splash of vodka

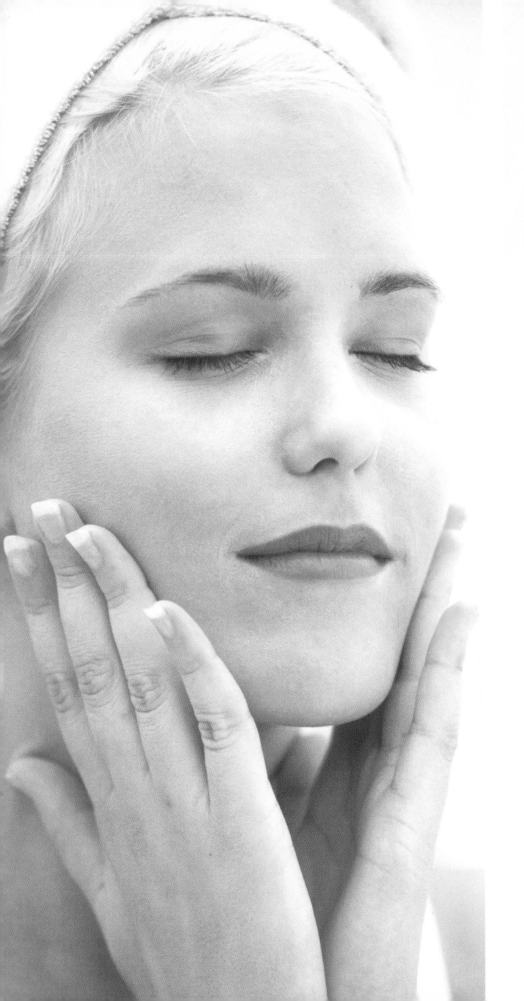
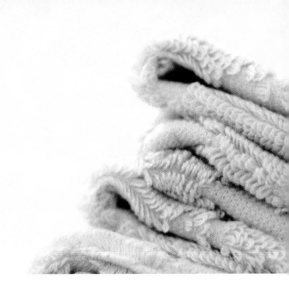

Stroking, kneading, pressing —
massage is the oldest healing method
in the world and yet it not only
helps to treat symptoms but in general
it also assists with the physical
feeling of well-being and mental
balance, bringing with it new
vitality and a zest for life. Massage
also helps you to rediscover your
own body and to get to know its
desires. When two people give
each other pleasure with a gentle
massage, they are meeting in a
very special intimate situation
in which they come close through
a shared experience in an almost
magical way and touch each other's
very souls.

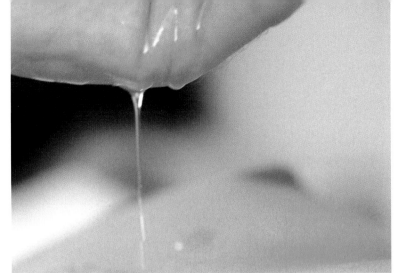
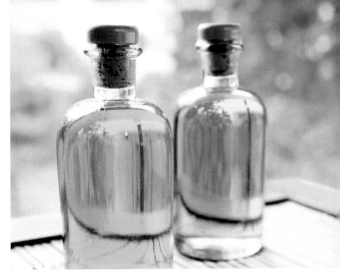

Massage:
The Art of Touching
Body and Soul

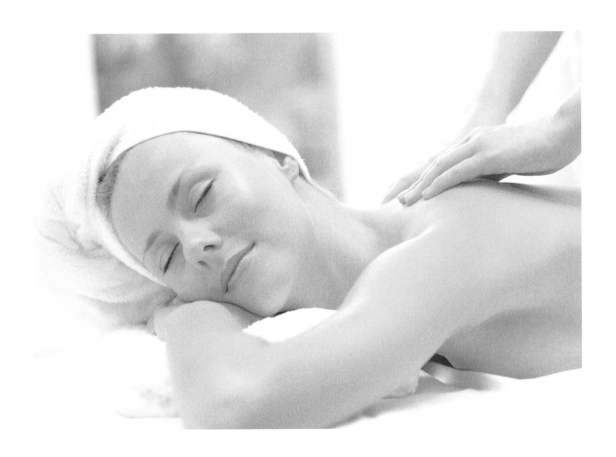

The Healing Power of the Hands

Massage is considered to be one of the world's oldest methods of healing. Ever since ancient times, people have repeatedly endeavoured to alleviate physical afflictions and to bring relaxation through touching, stroking and kneading. Each and every culture has developed its own methods and techniques. Traditions from China date back to the third millennium before Christ. In Ayurveda, the celebrated ancient Indian health philosophy, a significant role is attributed to the healing power of the hands. The Greeks and Romans also knew about the importance of massage in sport. In the western world, the best-known massage technique from ancient China is acupressure: in the same way that acupuncture uses needle pricks to produce certain effects, acupressure involves a series of pressure points in the body, which are stimulated to trigger irritation that brings about healing and well-being. The fundamental principles of today's classical massage were developed in Sweden in the 19th century.

The Art of Touching Body and Soul

In our modern culture, physical contact continues to play a subordinate role even today. Apart from a clearly defined north-south divide – in the south people are considerably warmer to each other, embrace each other and touch each other – we behave in a very reserved manner in our physical contact with others. Essentially, our contact is limited to shaking hands. You can definitely say that in our culture, the sense of touch is quite neglected in comparison with our other senses.

After all, touching is vital. Every human being has a primaeval yearning for physical contact. This begins in the first months of our lives. We know that frequent physical contact even helps babies with their physical development. Babies who experience plenty of physical attention increase in size and weight faster than children who miss out on it. And nowadays, you can learn a special baby massage aimed at giving children the pleasure of experiencing extensive contact.

We know too that a lack of physical contact can lead to psychological deficiencies and even depression. Old people are a good example – it is recommended that they get themselves a pet (best of all a dog or a cat),

Even for babies, special massage techniques have proved extremely beneficial.

which they not only have to care for but also can stroke. For the person doing the touching, the experience is as just as pleasant as for the one receiving the attention. Stroking is good for both of them.

Why do We Enjoy Massage?

Massage – treatment through touching – has a holistic effect that moves and arouses the entire body and the mind. Massage helps to regenerate the body and it supports and even challenges the self-healing powers – powers that lie within the capacity of every reasonably intact organism. Massage works by stimulating the skin through touching the nerve endings. It does not really matter whether you massage yourself or someone else massages you.

Massage stimulates the blood circulation and the lymph flow. Through massage, you can even influence the functioning of the internal organs such as the digestive system. You can massage the abdomen according to a particular method so as to have a beneficial effect on the intestinal system. Individual organs can be directly influenced through foot reflex zone massage, in which the various points on the sole of the foot correspond to particular organs.

Of course massage has an especially intensive effect on the nervous system, the sensors of which lie beneath the skin. One and the same massage manoeuvre can, depending on how it is carried out, have either a stimulating or a calming effect. In the case of muscular tension, massage works wonders. Systematic touching also has a more indirect effect: hormones are released which cause an intense feeling of happiness to stream through the entire body.

Even conventional medicine, in which nothing is validated until its effect can be unequivocally demonstrated, recognises the benefits of massage. Severe pain such as headaches, muscular and joint complaints and even cardiovascular infirmities, insomnia and digestive problems can be alleviated by using certain massage techniques.

Massage is a tried and tested remedy for alleviating stress conditions and tension. It can help invigorate and stimulate. Massage – and not just as manipulation involving a partner – can stimulate sexual desire. Everyone knows how good it feels when you stroke your hands, abdomen or face

Massage has a very positive effect that alleviates many health problems.

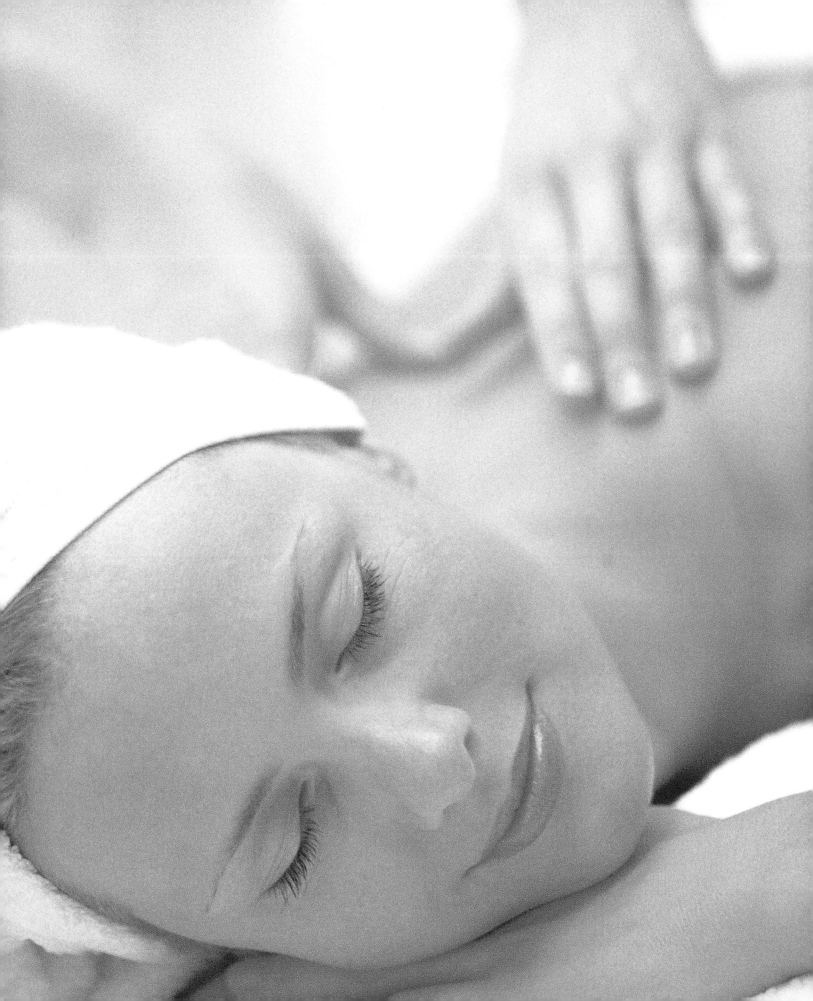

yourself. And massage makes you beautiful. By stimulating the blood circulation, massage can actually promote beauty by smoothing out wrinkles and relieving tension. The effect on beauty can, however, also be an indirect one: the physical contact of massage stimulates the whole body, lending wings to the imagination – and happiness makes you beautiful. But it is important to know that massage can really only help if you use it on a regular basis. A single massage session may be a very pleasant experience, but it will naturally not have lasting success. Massage only works if it is repeated at regular intervals – and of course this touching and being touched can be addictive. Ayurveda makes use of so-called synchronized massage, in which two masseurs treat the body in the same rhythm. The very thought of four hands moving over their back, arms and legs in synchronised rhythm puts some people in an extremely happy mood.

A MASSAGE IS NOT ALWAYS APPROPRIATE

Massage too has its limitations: in pregnancy, for example, massage can present problems. If you know which massage techniques are suitable, these can be bring considerable relief to the mother-to-be. But applied wrongly, massage can also have detrimental effects. In the case of serious cardiovascular problems, high blood pressure, heart attack, influenza and other feverish infections, phlebitis, varicose veins or if there is a risk of thrombosis, you should do without a massage or at least seek the advice of a doctor. For injuries or fresh scars, too, massage is of no advantage. The professional masseur is always aware of when he or she must show restraint and knows how to use his or her art sensibly in case of illness. But here we will only be dealing with the type of massage that anyone can practise, either alone or together with a partner.

OIL MAKES THE SKIN SUPPLE

You can massage without oil and cream. Of course, it makes sense to use oil, and you will not find any professional masseur who works without it. Why is this? By using oil, the hands become supple and glide almost playfully over the body. The person receiving the massage also experiences this as more pleasant than if dry hands were working on his or her body.

The body can absorb substances through the skin more rapidly than when they are taken as medication. Components of the oils can thus be detected in the blood only 20 minutes after they are applied to the skin.

Nor should you forget that certain vegetable oils have a caring, even healing effect on the skin.

Olive oil troubles many people because it smells too much like salad dressing. It is best to combine the intense smell with sesame oil, which is neutral and contains natural antioxidants. By the way, you should always use olive oil from the first press. Sweet almond oil nourishes the tissues and – except in the case of oily skin – is frequently used in view of its wide range of possible applications. Its smell is characteristically slightly sweet and nutty. Grapeseed oil saturates the skin without oiling it, and is also quite economical. Vitamin-rich, nourishing avocado oil should be mixed with a carrier oil because of its strong smell.

Two oils are indispensable not just for an effective massage but also for a simultaneous internal treatment: borage oil for dry skin and evening primrose oil for aging skin. Both oils have high proportions of linolenic and gammalinolenic acid. These are primary substances for the development of prostaglandin. As a central control element, prostaglandin is involved in numerous metabolic processes. It is effective against inflammation of the skin, prevents thromboses, helps people who are overweight and affords protection against arteriosclerosis. The only disadvantage of these highly saturated oils is that they quickly turn rancid. So make sure they are put into special bottles from which the oxygen can be extracted.

Coconut oil was originally brought to Europe from India. Here, it still numbers among the classics even today; it is mostly sold is solid form and has to be liquefied through heating. Essential ylang-ylang oil increases the skin's capacity for binding water. In South-east Asia, it is frequently used for hair care.

Jojoba oil, which has a long tradition as a tried and tested remedy of the North American Indians, is a good basic substance; however, it is not an oil in the classical sense but rather liquid wax. The advantage of this oil is that it does not oxidize and thus does not turn rancid. It is therefore the ideal oil for working in essential oils. It is a popular remedy for irritated skin, psoriasis and eczema.

Wheatgerm oil is squeezed from wheat seeds. It has a high proportion of amino acids, lecithin and the vitamins A, B, C and K. It enhances the skin's elasticity, creating a protective film and helping particularly in the case of tired skin.

Aloe oil contains numerous enzymes, trace elements, minerals and vitamins. As this oil stores moisture, which it releases on to the skin, it not only has a regenerating effect and retards the aging process but it also helps against sunstroke and burns.

There are also massage oils to which essential oils and other substances are added. In this way, not only is a pleasant scent produced but there is also a very differentiated effect on the body, as the essential substances penetrate into the skin to bring about some highly specific benefits.

THE MAGIC OF ESSENTIAL OILS

You can also use the massage oils we have mentioned here as a basis, i.e. as so-called carrier oils, to which you can add a few drops of essential oils as aromatic substances. But even these carrier oils contain important healing substances. The added fragrant substances make an additional contribution to the sense of well-being during the massage because of their bewitching scent, and they make you feel considerably better and have a positive effect on your state of mind. Aroma therapy systematically makes use of the healing effect of essential oils in order to overcome certain organic disorders.

Essential oils are extracts from seeds (e.g. coriander, caraway), roots (e.g. angelica, vetiver), wood (e.g. rosewood, cedar, sandalwood), resin

Be careful with essential oils. These highly concentrated liquids can cause serious irritation if they are applied to the skin undiluted. In particular, they must not get into the mucous membranes. One drop on the finger, only superficially washed off under water, can cause unpleasant irritation if you then rub your eye.

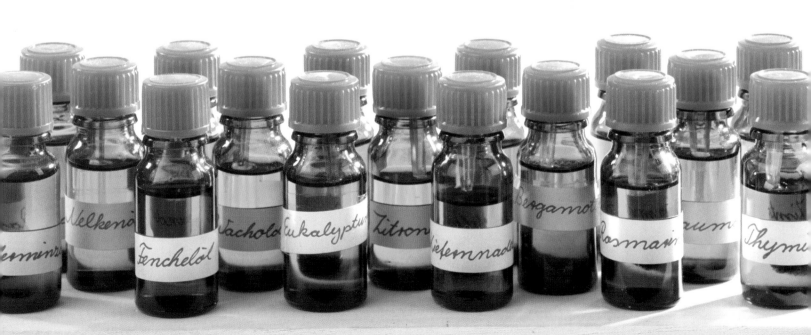

(e.g. benzoin, myrrh), fruit peel (e.g. citrus fruits) or bark (e.g. cinnamon). Essential oils are, as a rule, very expensive because huge quantities of plant matter are required to extract a mere fraction of an ounce of oil. On the other hand, these highly concentrated essences are also very rich and you only need to add a few drops of them to a mixture.

One of the best things about these oils is that you can mix them according to your own taste and thus devise individual scent creations. Mind you, you should not mix more than three oils together. As particular effects are attributed to each oil, you should of course ensure that you do not combine oils with conflicting effects. An oil that has an invigorating effect should not be combined with one to which a particularly calming effect is attributed.

ESSENTIAL OILS – INTENSIVE EFFECTS ON THE BODY

Essential oils, aromatic essences or aromatic oils are not fatty oils: their components, which largely volatile, do not stain paper.

Concentrated from primary or specific active ingredients, essential oils can provide a fast-acting therapy. The properties of a plant as an infusion, powder or concentrate are often different from the properties of the essential oils from the same plant. The oil geranium robert for example, which is not distilled, is said to have anti-diabetic properties. The essential oil of geranium bourbon, however, does not have this effect.

In view of thier rapid effects, three to six weeks (a maximum of three months) is generally enough to restore balance in the case of problems that are to be treated with aroma therapy.

Essential oils, regardless of which part of the body they applied to, are attracted by the area where there is a disorder of an organ or bodily function. This is a specific characteristic of essential oils. Plants and plant juices do not have this property.

There are only very few essential oils that can be used either alone or in a mixture without being diluted. All other essential oils have to at least be mixed with oil or diluted with wheatgerm, olive or calendula oil or a neutral body milk.

You can use the following oils undiluted: eucalyptus, geranium, ylang-ylang, cajeput tree, chamomile, pine, caraway, lavender, marjoram, niauli, orange, rosewood, rosemary, juniper, cedar, lemon, cypress and petit grain.

You can dilute the following oils with a carrier oil or mix them with another essential oil: green aniseed, basil, bergamot, verbena, tarragon, ginger, coriander, lemon grass, nutmeg, cloves, oregano, summer savoury, peppermint, bitter orange, rose, sassafras tree, turpentine, thuya, thyme and cinnamon. However, you should be particularly careful with peppermint, thyme, oregano and ginger because of the intensity of these oils.

Essential oils are not a universal remedy, but in numerous cases they relieve skin problems, have an effect on general well-being and result in a clear improvement in vital energy. This effect is already noticeable five to six days after a treatment.

When the Egyptians began to use essential oils not only for embalming corpses, but also for treating the living body, they did this by means of rubbing (embrocation). They highly valued not just the smell of the oils but also their healing properties. This gave rise to perfume – mixtures of essential oils to suit individual desires and tastes.

After an application of essential oils to the skin, traces of them can be detected in the blood and lymph after about four hours. Everyone can boost his or her vital capacity by rubbing in essential oils, thereby supporting the body's long-term ability to wake up in the morning and to relax and get good recuperative sleep in the evening.

There are different kinds of embrocation, such as a toning embrocation in the morning, or its counterpart, a relaxing embrocation in the evening. In the case of meals that are hard to digest, a special embrocation directed at the digestive system is recommended. Breathing and cardiovascular embrocations improve the cellular oxygen intake. There are, however, also embrocations for pain and even embrocations that stimulate sexual desire, making it possible to achieve astonishing sexual peaks.

Since children have very sensitive skin, you should always mix the embrocations for them with an equal share of wheatgerm, sweet almond or olive oil. Babies who have not yet reached the age of six months must not be treated with essential oils at all!

For an embrocation, use essential oils in the following quantities, diluted with a carrier oil:
Body: 30 drops
Stomach: 5–10 drops
Aches and pains: 5–10 drops
Legs: 5–20 drops
Hair: 50–100 drops
Face: 3–5 drops
Chest and back: 20–30 drops
Feet: 10 drops

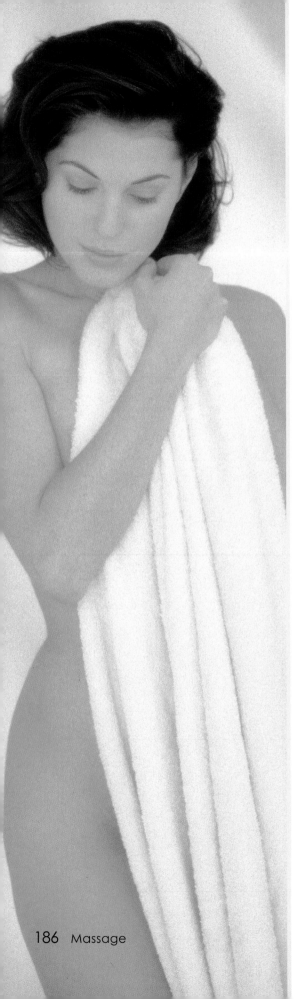

HOW TO CARRY OUT AN EMBROCATION

Put several drops of the selected mixture in the palm of your hand. Briefly rub your hands together and then spread the mixture over the parts of the body that are to be treated. Rub the oil in with slow clockwise rotating movements.

You should carry out toning and relaxing embrocations in the morning between 6 a.m. and midday, or in the evening between 6 p.m. and midnight. An embrocation with an aphrodisiac effect is best taken at about 5 p.m. or just before you go to bed. Embrocations for the digestion are carried out just after a meal. You can do embrocations for breathing in the mornings and evenings; for circulation it is recommended that they be done in the morning, at 5 p.m. or before going to bed. Foot embrocations can be carried out at any time of the day or night. Embrocations for the scalp and the face are likewise not subject to time constraints and are carried out for beauty and well-being.

To make it easier for your body to start the day, you should try out the following morning embrocation. First you have to venture under the cold shower, then breathe in and out slowly, deeply and evenly for a few minutes. Now put 20 to 30 drops of a tonic oil mixture on your chest, back, nape of the neck, spinal cord, the soles of your feet and your solar plexus. Always rub in the oil in a circular motion and in a clockwise direction. Set aside one and a half to two minutes every morning for this massage. The following oils, used in pure form, are suitable in the morning: geranium, pine, rosemary, rosewood, sandalwood, cedar and lemon. You have to dilute these essential oils with a carrier oil: verbena, oregano, nutmeg, coriander, summer savoury, peppermint, thyme or cinnamon.

For an evening embrocation you should first have a warm shower or a relaxing warm bath. Then do your breathing exercises for three minutes. Finally allow yourself a relaxing embrocation with 20 to 30 drops of essential oil plus the carrier oil – apply to your chest, back, nape of the neck, spine, the soles of your feet, arms, legs and the solar plexus.

Essential oils work not just through the skin but also through the sense of smell, and they have an internal effect. If you leave a small bottle open or spill a couple of drops, you will immediately notice the overpoweringly intensive smell. With the help of various utensils, you can also spread the smell of the oils throughout the room. You can obtain so-called aroma ventilators from specialised dealers. You drip the oils onto a cartridge, which you then insert into the device. The built-in ventilator whirls the scent around. Diffuser aerosol devices are also electrically operated; they spray the essential oils into the air in tiny droplets without warming them. These droplets in turn ionize microparticles suspended in the air in much the same way that in nature, the wind uses the sun's energy to distribute ionized oxygen in the atmosphere.

Thermal fragrance blocks are nothing more than electrical warming plates that heat the water dishes above them, causing the water and the oil contained in it to evaporate. Since nothing can burn with these devices, unlike fragrance lamps with candles, they are especially suitable for children's or elderly people's rooms.

However, this process can be carried out even more simply: in fact, any receptacle that can be filled with plenty of water will suffice. Put a couple of drops of the oils into it and place the vessel on a heat source such as a small stove. Fragrance lamps are generally more attractive, but they work in exactly the same way as a receptacle on the stove.

"Ceramic rings" are lamp rings made from non-glazed ceramics, on to which the essential oil mixture is applied in drops; the ring is screwed into the socket of an electric lamp. This is a particularly good solution if you are away from home but do not want to do without your usual aroma therapy. In this way, you can even enjoy it in the evening in your hotel room after a stressful day at a conference.

The most popular types of oil therapy are without doubt inhalation and the facial steam bath (as described in the chapter "200 bath essences for your well-being"). In the case of dry inhalation, you put essential oils on a handkerchief or ball of cotton wool and inhale them through the nose. This method is suitable for people who do not like hot vapours.

Oil Mixtures for Massage

Fragrant Oil for a Back Massage

10 ml ($^1/_3$ oz) diluted lavender oil
1 drop lemon grass oil
1 drop bergamot oil

Mix 10 ml ($^1/_3$ oz) of diluted lavender oil with a drop each of the two essential oils lemon grass and bergamot. This quantity is sufficient for a massage.

Anti-stress Oil

10 ml ($^1/_3$ oz) ylang-ylang oil
10 ml ($^1/_3$ oz) sweet almond oil
1 drop chamomile oil
3 drops pure lemon oil

Put 10 ml ($^1/_3$ oz) of diluted ylang-ylang oil into the same quantity of sweet almond oil and then enrich this mixture with a drop of essential oil of roman chamomile and three drops of pure lemon oil. This massage has a wonderfully relaxing effect.

Anti-pain Oil

10 ml ($^1/_3$ oz) unmodified olive oil
10 ml ($^1/_3$ oz) diluted juniper oil
2 drops black pepper oil
4 drops marjoram oil

If you suffer from aching joints or rheumatic pain, we recommend a special massage oil mixture that is highly popular in France. This oil is especially suitable for women suffering from dropsy, poor blood circulation, oily skin, acne or painful periods. The essential oil also has an effect on nervous conditions and is very beneficial in cases of anxiety.

Combine 10 ml ($^1/_3$ oz) each of unmodified olive oil and diluted juniper oil and enrich this mixture with two drops of black pepper oil and four drops of marjoram oil.

Anti-cellulite Massage Oil

10 ml ($^1/_3$ oz) diluted juniper oil
2 drops juniper oil
2 drops geranium oil
2 drops lemon oil

Mix 10 ml ($^1/_3$ oz) of diluted juniper oil as a carrier substance with the following essential oils – two drops each of juniper, geranium and lemon. As this mixture is suitable for the treatment of cellulitis, you should give a thorough massage involving plucking in accordance with Dr. Jacquet's method (as described on page 199) and then carefully massage this oil mixture into the skin.

ANTI-PAIN MACERATION

Maceration is a process in which materials are soaked so that the active ingredients are absorbed by the carrier substance. To make a maceration, take some flowers, cover them with twice their volume of carrier oil and leave to macerate in a closed container in a dark place for about a month.

For a special anti-pain maceration, use jasmine flowers and cold-pressed olive oil. Use the oil for a whole body massage after a relaxing bath or apply it to the reflex zones.

3 cups jasmine flowers
1 l (2 pints) cold-pressed olive oil

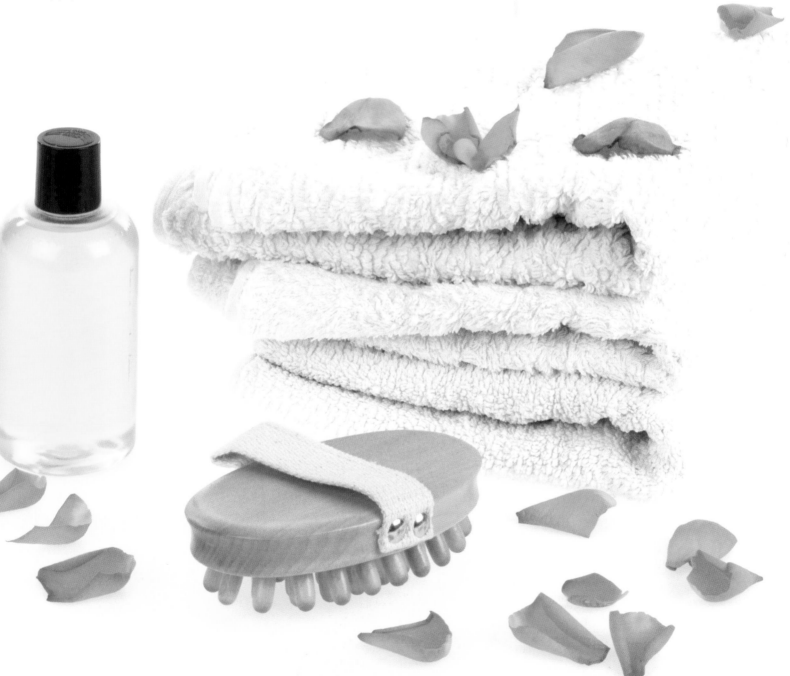

PREPARATIONS FOR THE MASSAGE

You can have a massage done while sitting or lying down, although many people find the latter more pleasant. If you are sitting down, you should choose a chair with a straight back on which you can sit in a relaxed manner.

If you want to give your partner a whole body massage, you will need a solid underlay because you can only massage the whole body in a lying position. In very rare cases you will, however, have a suitable couch at your disposal, just like the ones masseurs use. If you are using a sofa or the bed, the person doing the massage will have to bend fairly far down and this will not do him or her much good. Beds are also unsuitable for a massage because the mattresses are mostly too soft and give way too readily. However, it is best to massage your partner on the bed if you are doing it just before he or she goes to sleep.

The partner doing the massage should always be sure to adopt a relaxed position. It is also essential that he or she wear comfortable clothing.

However, you can also lie down on the floor. Pad the underlay somewhat, for example with a sleeping bag, futon, thin mattress, quilt, a mat made of foam material or with thick woollen blankets. For protection against the oils, the surface should be covered with large towels. A cushion or rolled-up towel makes for further comfort. Keep your back straight while you massage. You should use kneepads if you are kneeling on the floor.

How to Massage

We would like to make one thing clear: you do not need training as a professional masseur. Basically, massage is not difficult at all. When you "massage" yourself or your partner, you quite instinctively do it correctly in most cases. You stroke the skin, work the muscles – exactly as it pleases you or the other person. There can be no objection to this. But if you familiarise yourself a little with the basic techniques of massage, everything will work out even better.

It is worth noting a couple of basic rules. Fundamentally, you should always massage towards the heart, for example the arms from the hands to the shoulder or the legs from the tips of the toes to the thigh. You should not massage directly on bones or the spinal column, because that would feel very unpleasant. Stop massaging if it is hurting your partner. If you massage a tense muscle it certainly hurts, but at the same time it gives rise to a pleasant feeling of relief. However, if the feeling of pain is unpleasant, you must stop the massage, at least on the affected spot.

You can feel muscular tension. A relaxed muscle feels beautifully soft. A tense muscle, on the other hand, has hard spots and is painful when massaged.

Anyone who massages himself or herself should also get in the right mood for it physically and loosen up his or her body by means of circular movements with the head, stretching or diaphragmatic respiration.

As a rule, a professional full massage takes half an hour, but it can also be extended to a whole hour. For a feel-good massage for yourself or your partner, you should however not be excessive. Ten to fifteen minutes are completely sufficient. During this period, you can massage a particular part of the body intensively or massage from head to foot.

Try out the following basic manoeuvres on yourself first (although naturally not on your back), because you can then better judge for yourself how softly or strongly you can get to work on your partner.

STROKING

A massage always commences with stroking. This also creates the first physical contact with the person receiving the massage, gets the partners attuned to one another and also serves the purpose of distributing the massage oil or cream evenly over the skin. At the end of the massage, ensure a pleasant finale by stroking.

For stroking, place your pre-oiled hands (please do not use too much oil, otherwise it will no longer be possible to apply intensive pressure) flat on the body together (see illustration below left). Then slide upwards evenly, applying more or less strong pressure with the balls of the thumb, fan out and follow the contours of the body back with reduced pressure (see illustration below right). You can vary the speed. Slow, soft stroking has a relaxing effect. Faster stroking stimulates the blood circulation.

Circling is a variant of this. Simply move the palms of your hands in circles over the skin. This manoeuvre too has a relaxing and calming effect. To circle with both hands, put them flat on the body some distance apart. Your hands then glide in a wide arc over the body and finally join again to form a circle.

KNEADING

When kneading, work the muscular tissue almost as if you were kneading dough. Take up a part of the muscle with your thumb and index finger and

Throughout the massage, you should always maintain physical contact with your partner with one hand. If you were to lift both hands, the overall relaxed mood would be interrupted and perhaps even destroyed. Therefore always massage in a flowing, even rhythm and never with broken or abrupt movements.

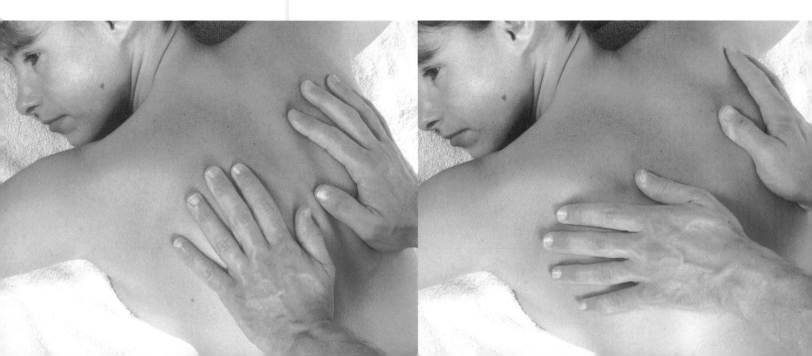

roll, press and push (see illustration below left). For this, the skin should neither be dry nor too oily: you could squeeze the muscles if there is excess oil or you could slide because it is too slippery. Intensive kneading promotes blood circulation, relieves tension and ensures that waste products are removed from the area being massaged.

PRESSING

The muscles are pressed together firmly with one or both hands, always in the direction of the muscular fibres in an upward movement towards the heart. You can apply the pressure either with your thumb or the palm of your hnad. But be careful: do not press too hard, and be sensitive – especially with the joints.

RUBBING

When rubbing, apply pressure to individual muscles by making small circling or spiralling movements with the tip of your thumb or the tips of your fingers (see illustration below right). Rubbing has a very relaxing effect.

PUMMELLING

Pummelling is a very particular technique. With the edge or palm of your hands, with your fists or with your cupped hands, make rhythmic chopping,

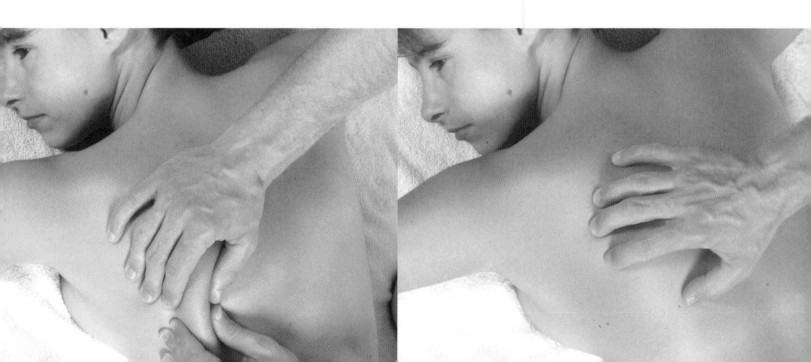

Give the forehead a wonderfully soft pressure massage:
With the backs of your hands, stroke the tension and folds out of the forehead. Place both hands on the side of the head and bring your thumbs together in the centre of the forehead. Move your thumbs outwards with slight pressure.

tapping, clapping and drumming movements. But be careful: never apply this technique on bones. Pummelling stimulates the blood circulation of the tissue and rouses your whole body.

A GENTLE HEAD AND FACE MASSAGE

A massage of this kind is wonderfully relaxing and can be full of tenderness. As a massage technique, you should use mostly stroking and circling movements here. But you can also knead your partner's eyebrows, cheeks and ears very gently. For massaging, it is best for you to sit or kneel behind your partner.

If you are working on the face with oil, please be very sparing with it. Make sure not to use essential oils, because these must not get into the eyes under any circumstances. On your partner's face, you can also do without oil altogether.

RELIEF FOR THE ARMS AND HANDS

The hands are the parts of the body that are the most active, so a little massage will be particularly good for them. First work on one arm and then on the other. Begin with the hand and work up to the shoulder. With the exception of the joints, you can work somewhat more strongly on the forearm and upper arm, kneading and pressing.

You can also loosen up the inside of the forearm by pressing and kneading. Massage the muscles between the fingers by smoothing out with both thumbs, from the fingers to the wrist. The palms of the hands are also worked with stroking and spiral-shaped rubbing movements of the thumbs towards the wrist.

NAPE OF THE NECK AND BACK

Most people find that their shoulders and the nape of the neck are tense. If feeling good and regeneration matter to us, a massage of the nape of the neck and shoulders is particularly important. Note how you react when you are in a tiring work posture: many people unconsciously massage the nape of their neck themselves from time to time.

First gently rub the nape of your neck and your shoulders. To relieve tension, really strong kneading is essential. (But be careful if there are any problems with the cervical vertebral column!) Rubbing and pressing are appropriate too. However, you should be careful: if the treatment hurts, then it is too strong and can even lead to headaches. So the dosage of the massage has to be just right. As long as the person being massaged feels good, you are doing everything correctly.

A back massage is absolutely wonderful. You can be more generous with the use of oil on the back, although the skin should of course not glisten with it. First spread the oil by gently stroking it on your partner's back. Then rub the back up and down lightly with large sweeping movements. Loosen up the back muscles by massaging more intensively; rubbing in circles or spiral movements frees up hard muscles. Finish by gently massaging the whole back.

INVIGORATE THE LEGS AND FEET

The legs have to carry the entire weight of the body. A particularly large amount of stress is placed on them through long periods of standing, unsuitable shoes and exertion during sport. There is nothing better for overtired legs than an extensive massage! And even if your legs do not ache, you will enjoy a loving massage as the highlight of your little feel-good programme.

First of all treat the back of both legs, then the front. The partner being massaged therefore lies first on his or her stomach and then turns over. The massaging movements are directed towards the heart. On the legs you can use all massage techniques, beginning with gentle stroking and then progressing to rubbing, pressing and kneading. Be careful with the knee joints! If your partner suffers from varicose veins or lymphatic oedema, i.e. water retention in the legs, you should leave massage to an expert.

Treat your partner's feet by pressing, stretching and pulling them. First massage one foot and then the other. Work first on the sole of the feet and then the insteps. Remember to massage the toes, as well as the spaces between them. Many people are very sensitive and ticklish on the underside of their feet. However, you can mostly control this by massaging more slowly and firmly.

THE ART OF SELF-MASSAGE

Used appropriately, self-massage can bring great relief. Try it and start the day with exhilaration, return to work with new strength after a short massage break or bring a stressful day to an end with a feeling of deep relaxation in the evening.

Many people tend to regard self-massage as a mere stopgap measure: you massage yourself simply because there is no one else around to do it. This may well be true, but you should remember that no one knows your body as well as you do yourself. Everyone knows himself or herself best, where he or she is feeling tension or how strongly the pressure needs to be applied to the skin and exactly which particular parts of the body need special attention.

Sometimes it is a good idea in between times to simply treat yourself to an invigorating five-minute massage – maybe at work when you are tired and worn out, on a boring trip in the bus or when you are sitting for hours in a cramped position on board a plane. In situations such as these, you can achieve an outstanding effect even with a self-massage, whether it be to invigorate or to relax you. All you need for this are your hands.

Massaging your back presents some difficulties; you need a partner for this. But with your face, the nape of the neck, with your chest and abdomen, hands, legs and feet, massaging yourself is no problem. You can even give yourself a whole body massage. For this, keep to a set sequence: begin with the feet, then go via the legs to the lower body and finally to the chest. Your head comes last.

WHAT CAN YOU ACHIEVE WITH A SELF-MASSAGE?

In the mornings it is probably important to you to banish all traces of tiredness so you can be fit to face the day ahead. The goal here is to get the organism going. When you massage yourself at work, on a long journey or in a monotonous waiting situation, you will want to do something about your tense muscles or perhaps just find some relief from stress in general. You can achieve outstanding success with a self-massage. In the evenings you will want to rid yourself of the stress of the day, the mental tension, so as to be fresh to enjoy a concert or a party. The massage techniques that need to be applied will help you achieve these goals. Circling and stroking movements, for example, have a very relaxing, calming effect and rid you of tension. Kneading and pummelling, on the other hand, will arouse and invigorate you.

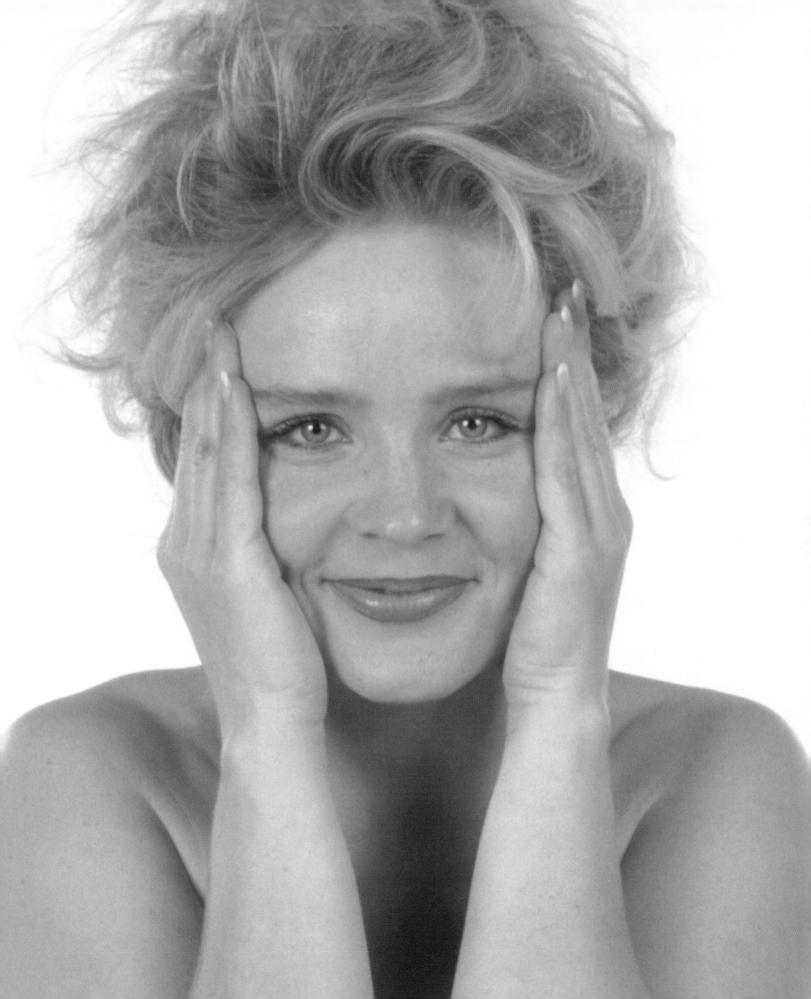

You do not need to undress to enjoy the comforts of a massage in between times. But you should try to withdraw a little, because you will rarely feel relaxed if a lot of people are watching you. You should at least adopt a comfortable posture. You can sit down on a sturdy chair with a firm seating surface and a straight back, or on a carpet on the floor, or better still on an exercise mat. If you are alone at home, you should simply take off your clothes and give your body the feeling of being completely free. In such cases, you should also use massage oil, as this will greatly increase your enjoyment. Your skin will feel the oil and its ingredients as a relief, and the fragrance that rises to your nose also has a positive effect on your olfactory sense.

THE FACE

A facial massage has an invigorating effect. It can drive away headaches, tiredness, nervousness and tenseness. And it also has a cosmetic effect. You can do a facial massage practically anywhere, and it won't take too long either. You only need to spare ten minutes in the morning, at work or in the evening. Use only a very small amount of oil for the facial massage; a teaspoon is quite sufficient. An oil such as almond oil is very suitable. A popular additive for the facial massage is rose oil. Stroking and gentle

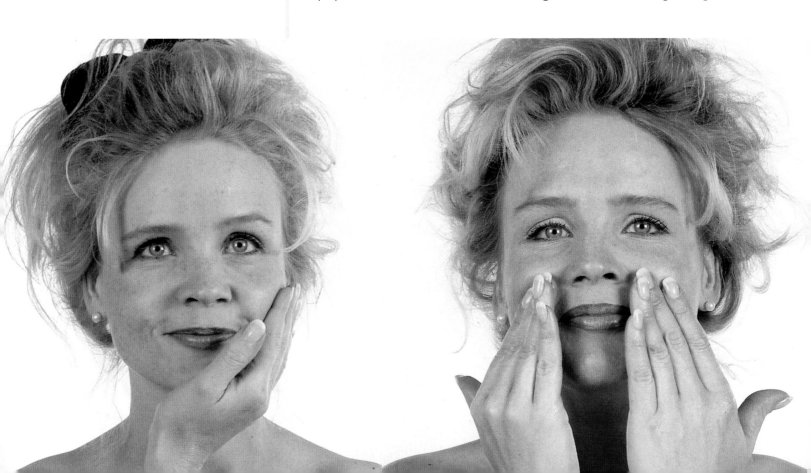

pressure are the techniques most commonly used. A morning facial massage is aimed above all at invigorating you, so this calls for rapid, sweeping movements. In the evening, when you prefer a relaxing effect, calm, gentle techniques are more appropriate.

Gentle stroking with both hands at the beginning of the facial massage enhances relaxation (see illustration below far left). Circling, along with slight kneading movements beside the nose down to the chin, relieves tension in the face (see illustration below centre). Small circling movements with the fingertips over the forehead and temples have a calming effect (see illustration below).

Dr. Jacquet's Plucking Massage

This massage technique was first presented in 1907 at the Medical Faculty in Paris. For about fifteen years, it was used exclusively by doctors. Later, this technique was also taught by massage and cosmetics schools. Its true advantage is the amazing effect it achieves without the use of great force. Among other uses, this technique is considered to be especially successful for acne and cellulitis, and naturally it also increases general well-being in a quite extraordinary manner.

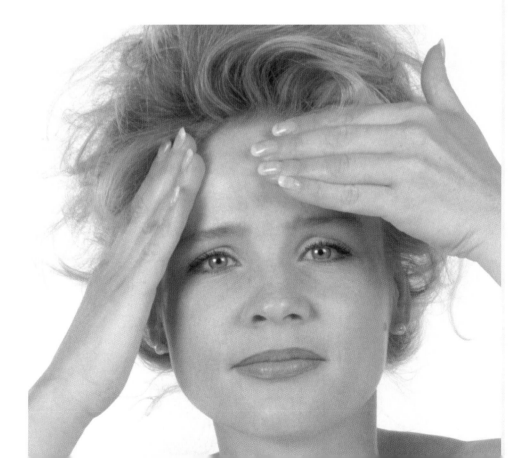

Mind you, you will have to do a fair bit of preparation. First soap your hands carefully and disinfect them with 70% alcohol. The nails must be quite short and the face pre-cleansed so that it is free of oil. Spray some refreshing sea water on to your face. Then cleanse the skin again with sea sediment exfoliation. The massage can now begin.

Briefly lift up the skin with all five fingertips without stroking, pummelling or turning, and then let go again straight away. You should never push the skin back and forth. Always begin in the middle of the face and move outwards. Pull rather slowly at first, but then do not be afraid to become more vigorous. On the forehead and on the nose, pick up the skin from the bony tissue using only your thumb, index finger and middle finger. On the face, neck and body, on the other hand, pluck with all five fingers. The important thing to remember is that every plucking movement has to be very short.

The Nape of the Neck

If you have no one to massage away the tension that you will often find in the shoulders and the nape of the neck, just do it yourself. You only need your hands and do not even have to get undressed for this treatment, so you can also use this technique at the office. You can massage the nape of your neck comfortably in a sitting position. This involves stroking at first; you then press and knead harder and finish off by stroking gently once more. To loosen up the muscles of the nape of your neck really well, move upwards to the base of the skull with circling movements of the thumbs. Close both hands around your neck and move forwards in the direction of your shoulders.

The Stomach

Whatever form of stomach ache you may be suffering from, a gentle massage will invariably bring relief. For the stomach massage, it is best to lie down on your back with your legs slightly bent. Move your hands in a circular motion and in a clockwise direction, and apply slight pressure to this area. It is important that the movement is not uninterrupted; it can also involve the whole of the upper body. Both hands can be used together, or one hand can circle in a clockwise direction around the navel with light, even pressure.

The Hands

Day after day, your hands have to perform really hard work. They become especially worn out doing professional tasks like typing on a computer for long periods. Massage the hands with stroking movements, rubbing, stretching and pulling. With firm pressure, rub the back of the hand with your thumb, moving upwards to the wrist. Follow this with strong circular movements of the thumb on the front of the forearm.

The Legs and Feet

Occupations which involve long periods of standing make for tired legs in the course of the day. And after sport, you can develop muscular cramp in the calf; warming up is good for the muscles before playing any kind of sport. It is therefore useful to know how to massage your own legs and feet. It is easier to massage a foot when you are sitting down with one leg crossed over the other. One hand supports the foot, and the other is free to perform the massage. Press along the middle of the sole of your foot with firm movements. Each toe is massaged individually by rolling, pressing and pulling.

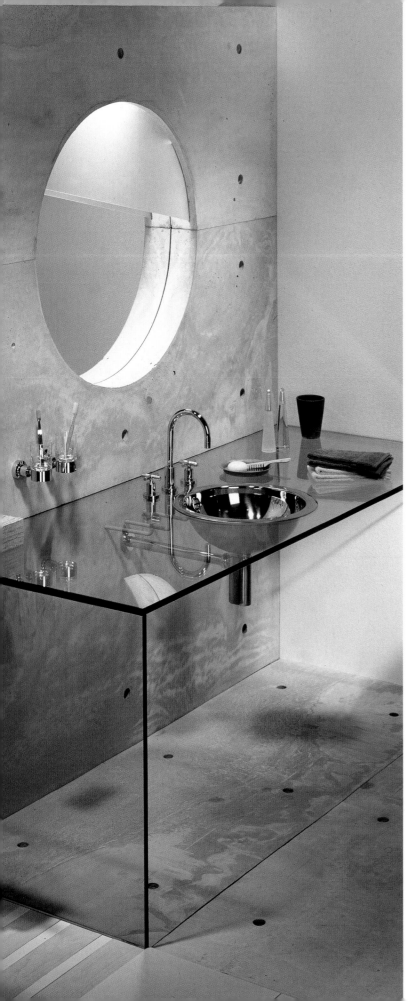

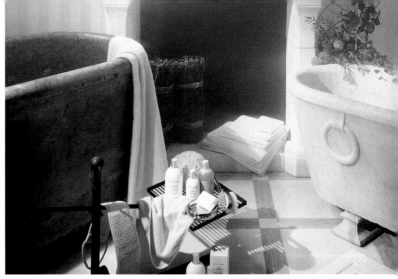

Whether you feel really good when taking a bath certainly depends on the makeup of the environment. It is no fun taking a bath in a tiny bathroom – one where it is obvious straight away that people only occasionally shower or clean their teeth in it, using it instead as a temporary dumping ground for all manner of things and as a place to dry their washing. The bathroom does not have to be luxurious or especially large: with imagination you can, even if only to a modest extent, create an inspiring basis for your personal bath festival. Of course if you are renovating anyway, you should make the most of this opportunity to set up an ideal bathroom for yourself. But even with minor corrections, with new tiles, with the astute use of colours and accessories, you can change an old bathroom around to such an extent that it is hardly recognisable.

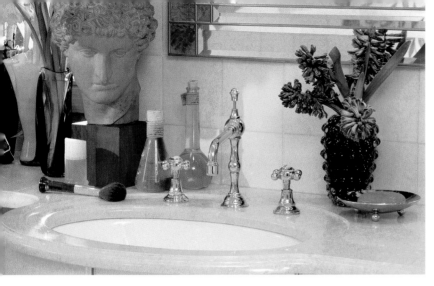
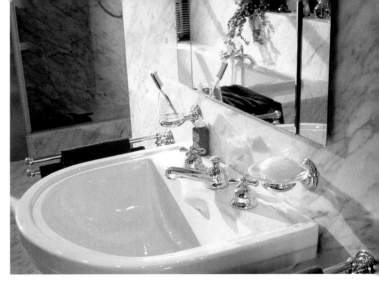

Your Own Bathroom:
An Oasis of Well-being

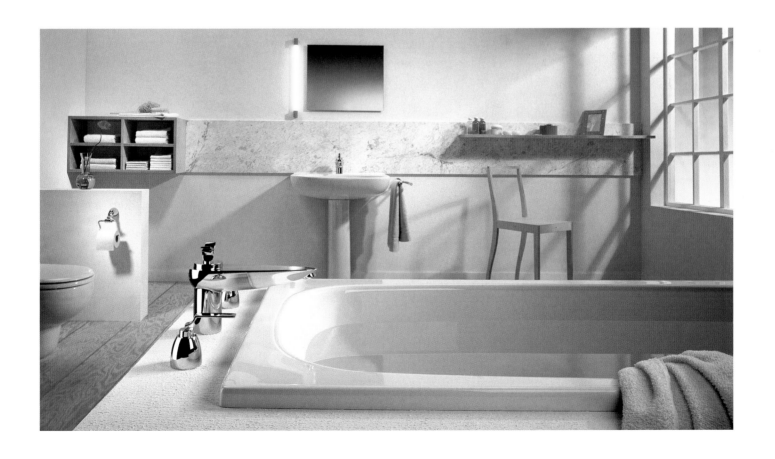

A PLACE FOR BODY AND SOUL

In this day and age, the bathroom is normally the smallest room in a home. In houses built a hundred years ago, however – if the architect conceded them a bathroom at all – an astonishing amount of space was accorded to this room. Obviously at that time the bathroom was held in high regard, at least in the more well-to-do circles, as a place for relaxation and recuperation. In the decades to follow, this awareness was lost and in the newly built homes bathrooms, like toilets, were mere necessities to which people paid no particular attention from an aesthetic point of view; people preferred to crowd the bath and the toilet together in a single room. Even homeowners, who basically could have done as they pleased regarding the size of their bathrooms, adhered to the unwritten principle that for purposes of hygiene as little space as possible should be squandered on a bathroom – unless, of course, the home in question was a particularly stylish, spacious villa.

THE BATHROOM IS REDISCOVERED

The age of the small bathroom that was limited to the role of a "wet cell" has long since passed. In our day and age, most of us value the bathroom as a room for personal recuperation and relaxation. In a home 100 square metres (1,000 square feet) in size – and this would almost be considered large by today's standards – there is of course only a little space left for a really generously dimensioned, beautiful bathroom. Nevertheless, size is not so crucial in this regard.

Naturally it is wonderful if you can position a large tub in the middle of the room, surround it with two washbasins and a bidet and still have room for a dresser and separate shower. A dream bathroom such as this, however, well and truly takes up as much space as would normally be available for a lounge. It is a dream, of course, but what do you do in reality? Most people move into an apartment or a house where the bathroom is a *fait accompli*. You simply have to come to terms with the way things are: whatever reservations you may have towards this room, you are left with the exisiting fittings, the wall tiles or the bathtub, since for practical reasons you first want to invest in renovating the rest of the home. That is understandable, too; after all, you do not live in the bathroom. The kitchen,

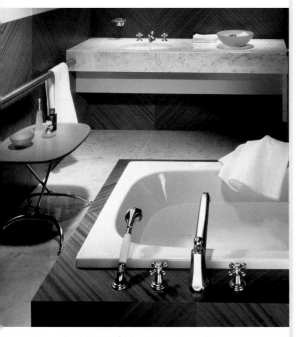

An elegant bath with clear lines and superior materials or a splendid bathing temple – there are no limits to the design and layout of your bathroom.

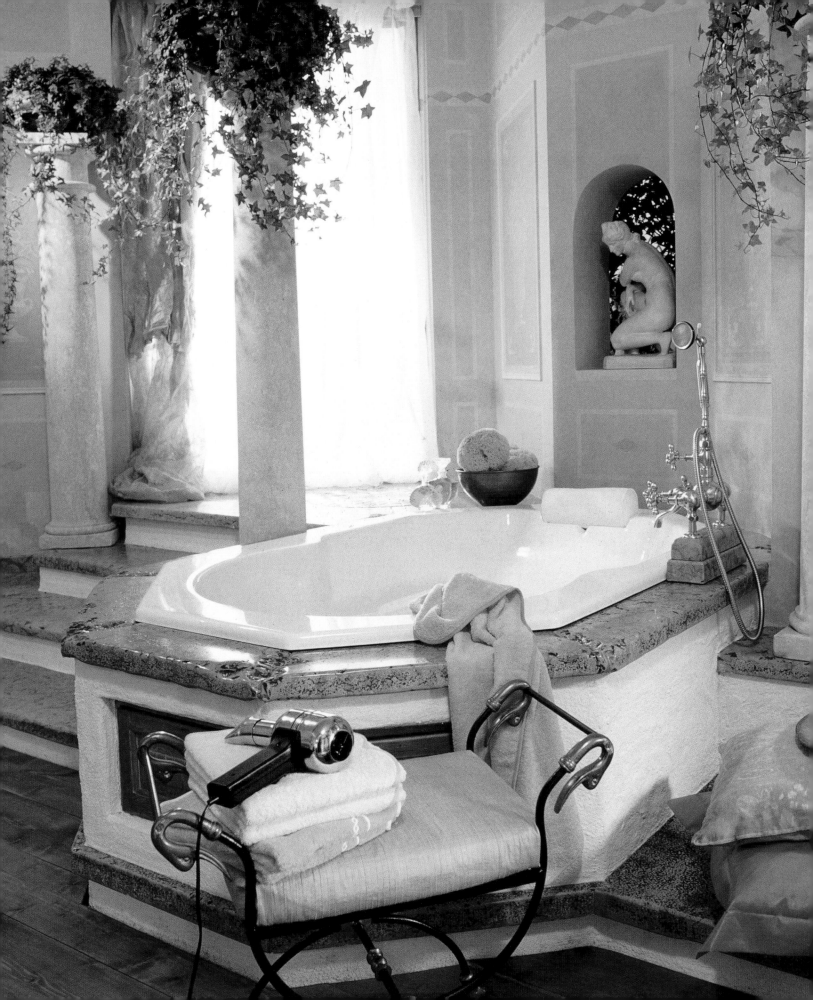

the living room, the children's room, perhaps even the bedroom – all of these have to be decked out as a matter of top priority. In addition, all the rooms apart from the bathroom are to a certain extent public: guests and friends spend most of their time there, whilst they only visit the bathroom or guest WC for a few minutes.

On the other hand, this does not mean that you cannot transform your existing bathroom into a personal paradise of well-being. If you decide to renovate the bathroom from scratch, do not simply choose any banal solution, but consider precisely what you can do with the space available. Anyone who thinks about it a bit will often come up with breathtaking solutions for creating, for example, an impression of generous spaciousness even in the smallest of rooms through the association of colours and shapes. And good ideas do not always have to be expensive. A costly large bathtub does not by any means lend a bathroom charm and magical powers. On the contrary, an ostentatious item like this could possibly destroy the balance of the room completely, whereas a better value tub that is also more modest in its proportions may fit much more favourably into the ambience.

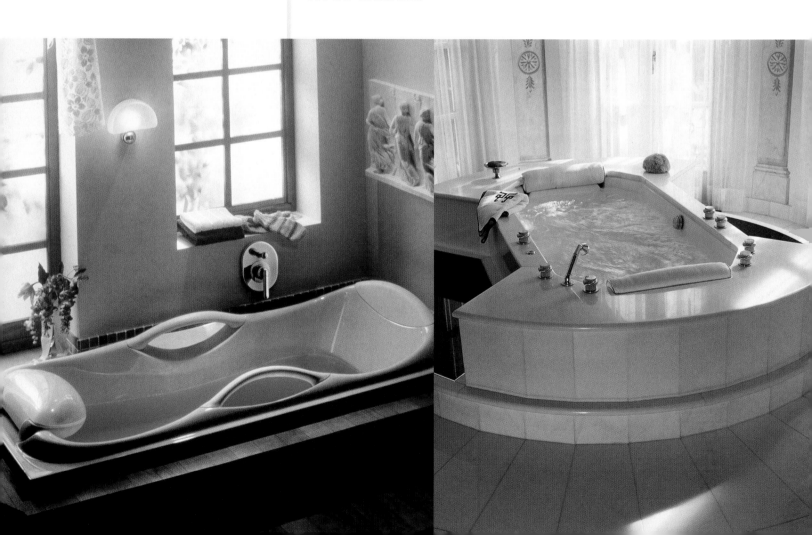

Perhaps you will choose to leave the old tub, the wash basin and the fittings where they are and you might first consider how you can give your bathroom – with freshly painted walls, a new floor, colours to match, a curtain, sophisticated lighting and accessories of all kinds – the style it needs for you to feel a sense of well-being.

Light is Life

If an excessively cost-conscious approach was adopted in the original planning of the bathroom, it is often not only the spatial circumstances that give cause for dismay: the window, too, is often very small. In such cases you must pay particular attention to installing adequate electric lighting. Electrical illumination is however also important for other reasons as well. As a rule, fluorescent lights are installed in bathrooms. They supply the room with light without sharply defined shadows; this, however, tends to destroy a pleasant atmosphere. If you must use fluorescent lights, you should at least choose tubes of a warm colour. White light has a cold effect and destroys all feeling and sensuality.

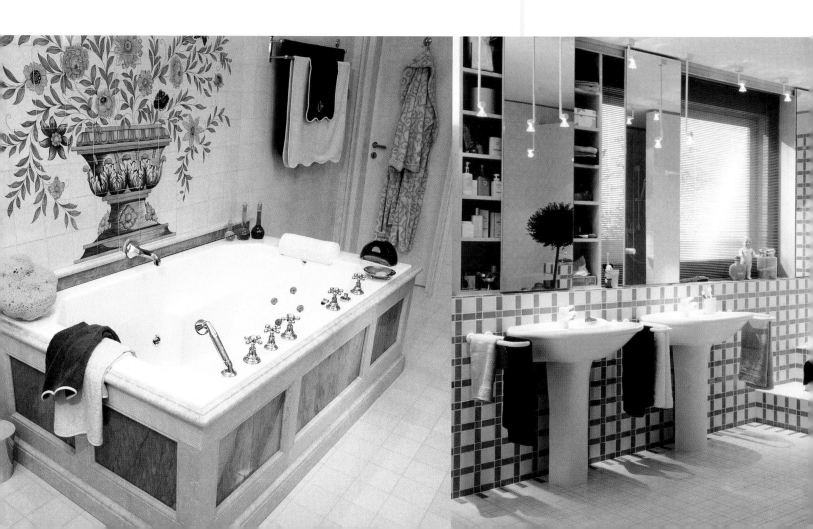

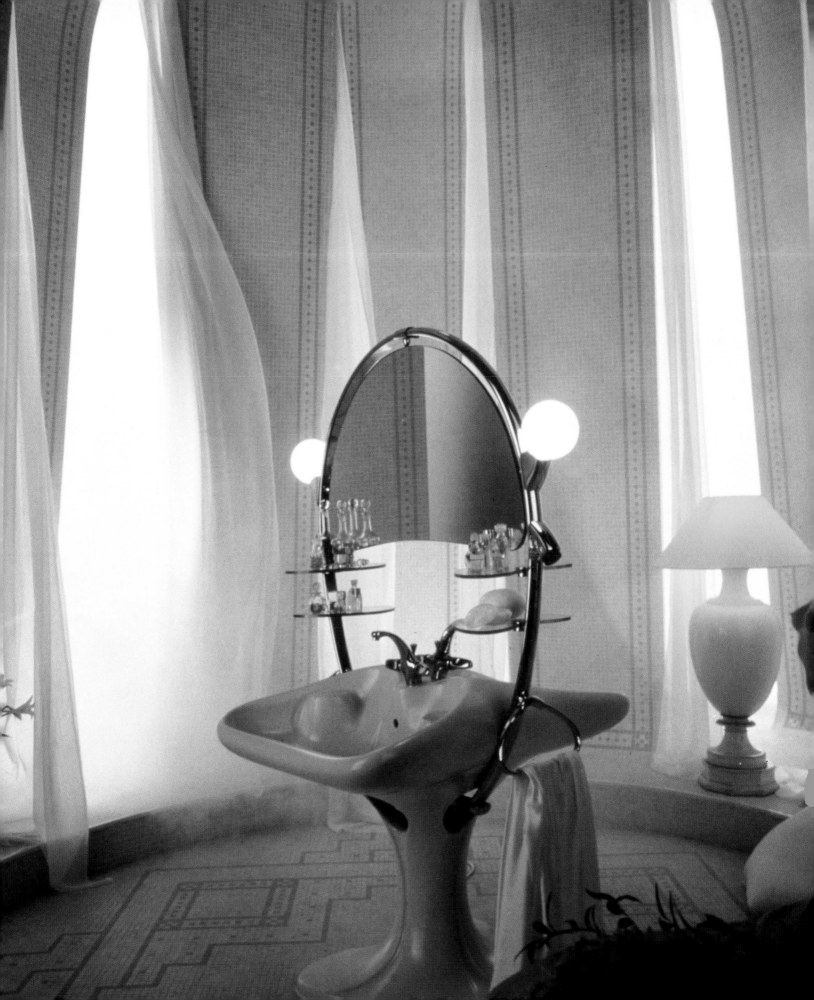

Halogen spotlights set into the ceiling that light up the whole room evenly although not in a sterile way are a good solution. Mirror cabinets are often also equipped with lamps and they supplement the light from above. However, you should, as a matter of principle, always get an expert to install all the electrical connections in the bathroom, rather than trying to do it yourself. Electricity and water side by side in a room like this can be a hazardous combination!

IF YOU ARE PLANNING A NEW BATHROOM

If you are in the fortunate position of being able to refit your bathroom from scratch, make good use of this opportunity and do it prudently. You must never be resigned to the way things are. To every bathroom problem there is a solution. The industry has now developed a range of the most sophisticated bathtubs, showers and washbasins of all sizes and shapes that makes it perfectly possible to fit out an original bathroom even if there is very little space available.

If the water and electrical connections have to be redone, you should come to an agreement with the tradespeople that a couple of reserve connections be provided to facilitate any adjustments to the bathroom that may become necessary in years to come as a result of changed situations. Above all you should not be stingy with electrical connections. The fact that a single socket over the washbasin is inadequate will be noticeable at the latest when you repeatedly have to pull out the plug from the shaver or the electric toothbrush in order to use your hair dryer. A strip with three or four sockets does not cost much more but will save you a lot of trouble every day. Never use double plugs and extension leads in the bathroom – that can soon become highly dangerous.

If you do not want to rip up all the walls when you are haveing the plumbing installed, you can have the pipes laid in front of the wall. They are first insulated for sound and heat and then lined. Finally the tiles are laid on top of the lining.

For the overall impression, it is crucial, especially for small bathrooms, that you select the right floor and wall covering. In small rooms you should dispense with dark colours. They would make the room seem even smaller and give you a stifling feeling. Light colours, on the other hand, make a

The modern bathroom would be unthinkable without electricity. Nevertheless, the electrical connections should be installed by an expert in such a way as to give off as little electromagnetic radiation as possible. Special cables with a high degree of shielding are commercially available for this purpose.

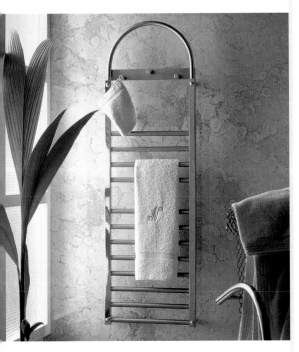

Modern heaters do not just ensure pleasant temperatures in the bathroom – they also serve as practical towel holders and warmers.

small room feel as if it has more generous proportions. Mirrors are not just there for you to have a good look at yourself; they also catch the light and give a room the impression of spaciousness.

Designing a windowless bathroom in such a way that you do not feel as if you are being constantly reminded of this limitation, and so that it is also a place where you really like to be, is a special challenge. As a rule, a single fluorescent tube over the mirror cabinet is not sufficient. You should consider whether additional halogen spotlights astutely set in a couple of inches into the ceiling might not convey the impression of a bright, congenial mood – as if the daylight were streaming in. Even the choice of the colour of the light is crucial and must of course be coordinated with the colours of the walls and the floor. In a windowless room, mirrors play an important role because, carefully positioned, they feign space even where there is hardly any at all.

Small bathrooms easily give the impression of being overcrowded if you keep your usual assortment of bath and washing implements there. The rudimentary small white cupboards that often used to be found under washbasins have now been superseded by imaginitive bathroom furniture available in all colours, sizes and shapes. These little space-saving wonders give you sufficient room for towels, soaps and shampoo bottles as well as being eye-catching. Nowadays you can also buy mirror cabinets in the most varied of designs, and their practicality is not readily apparent at first glance. On the outside they present themselves as elegant or oddly futuristic, but on the inside they boast a lot of space.

HIGH TECH IN YOUR BATHROOM PARADISE

Many people just shrug their shoulders when spa baths or fitness showers are discussed; after all, these fittings are still very expensive even by today's standards. But if you are renovating your bathroom from scratch, you should consider whether it might perhaps pay to invest in such an item after all. A spa bath – you can also purchase smaller cheaper models – is no mere technical gadgetry; it offers you the chance to regularly enjoy hydrotherapy.

Hydromassage with heat and air has a calming effect on the entire body, stimulates the immune system, brings the cardiovascular system into balance and has a general invigorating effect. Technology today also has something to offer the spa bath at home: this ranges from the soft air bubbles that swirl about the body to the strong water jet that massages muscles thoroughly. The jets built into the tub also give the body buoyancy so that you almost have the feeling of being borne aloft.

In technical terms, the hydro wonder works as follows: a blower presses the heated air through the jets into the tub. A sophisticated combination of jets, which are also adjustable, makes it possible then to choose between gentle tingling and a brisk massage jet. The tubs are designed in such a way that various jets at the side, in the region of the back and feet, give the body optimal care with the healing swirl of water.

Nowadays, even the once so humble shower can offer a complete fitness program. These facilities often also have room for two people and you can enjoy the wonders of water on a seat that folds down. The water does not just come from above but from all sides, and you can adjust the strength of the water jet.

Various applications can be activated and set via a display. In this way, you can, for example, enjoy a carefree alternating shower – without constantly having to fiddle about with the cold and hot taps. Some models even include a steam bath option. And of course an audio system is part of the luxury of bathing: you can listen to the music of your choice from a CD that you have put in beforehand.

TASTES VARY

There are countless options for fitting out and equipping a bathroom. Here too, beauty is in the eye of the beholder. And imagination knows no bounds. If you find yourself not wanting to leave your bathroom and get back to real life, you know that you have been successful in the design of your bathroom.

Many people prefer highly imaginitive nostalgic designs and choose tiles with rich ornamentation, fancy contoured fittings and mirrors with extravagant gilded frames and animal patterns. The bathtub can be made of enamelled cast iron with intricate borders and stand uncovered on clawed feet – and why not illuminate the entire scenario with the diffused light of tulip-shaped lamps?

A bathroom can be modified quite effectively even with frugal decorations

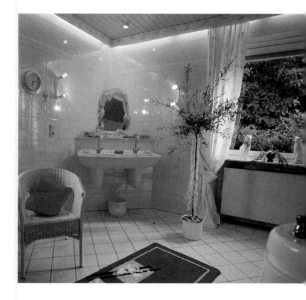

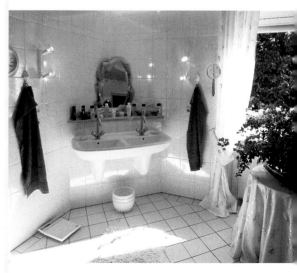

A bathroom in the country house style has its own cheerful, bright character. Tiles with floral patterns, airy light curtains, pretty corner shelves with an orchid in a ceramic pot, rustic taps and shower combination taps made of chrome or bronze, decorative empty bottles: these are the typical elements of this style. If you put furniture in the bathroom – high or low cupboards, chairs or stools – you should choose wooden ones, waterproof them and paint them in light pastel shades. Avoid modern accessories – the appearance should be somewhat weathered and faded with coarse surfaces, not streamlined. Acrylic plastic and chrome have no business here. You can for example store cakes of soap, sponges and massage towels in a wire basket formerly used for fetching eggs from the market. Perhaps you can position an aluminium milk canister in the corner. It can be fun rummaging through second-hand shops and visiting flea markets to look for the accessories you need.

It is stylish to paper the walls with waterproof wallpapers in bright congenial floral patterns. But if you insist on tiles, get ones without a fashionable design – perhaps just white or with a discreetl floral pattern.

Today, people who prefer clear lines have a huge range of tubs, washbasins and furniture to choose from. The elegance of this style is based on simplicity and functionality. However, quite a number of accessories can be ruled out right from the start. Consider carefully whether you want to

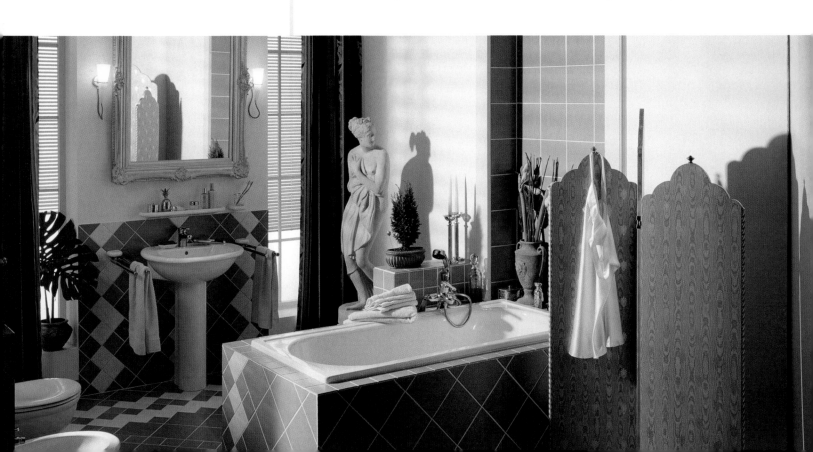

set a particular tone here or there with a vase or bowl. Windowsills and other surfaces where objects can be deposited or cupboards crammed full of sundry items would ruin the clear functional line of a modern bathroom landscape such as this.

When You Get Tired of Your Bathroom

The more special the style of bathroom you choose, the more you might, however, create some problems for yourself: what initially seems quite charming becomes boring after a while. You can change a curtain easily enough, but an expensive cast enamel bath with Baroque decoration embellishment. Of course nothing lasts forever, but hardly anyone will want to pay for new bathroom plumbing equipment every couple of years. However, as much as you may love extravagant things, you should be aware of the effects of wear and tear. So ask yourself quite candidly whether you will still like a particular combination in a few years' time. People find many styles captivating – for a certain time, and then they get tired of looking at them.

There is nothing to say that a neutral style has to be lacking in imagination. The basic equipment, consisting of the bathtub and washbasin, floor co-

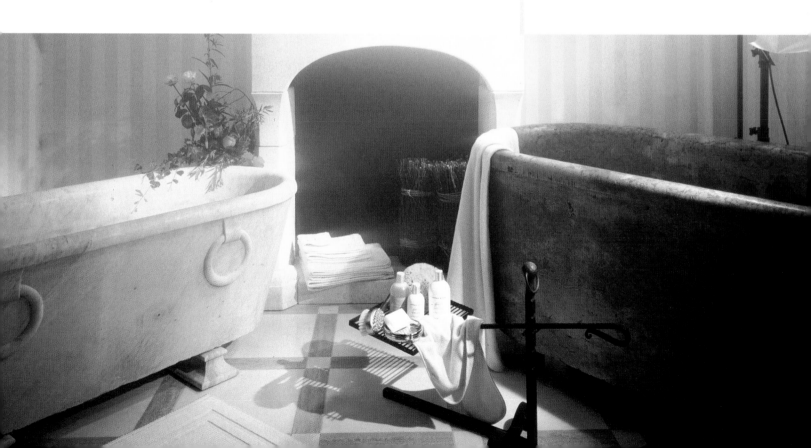

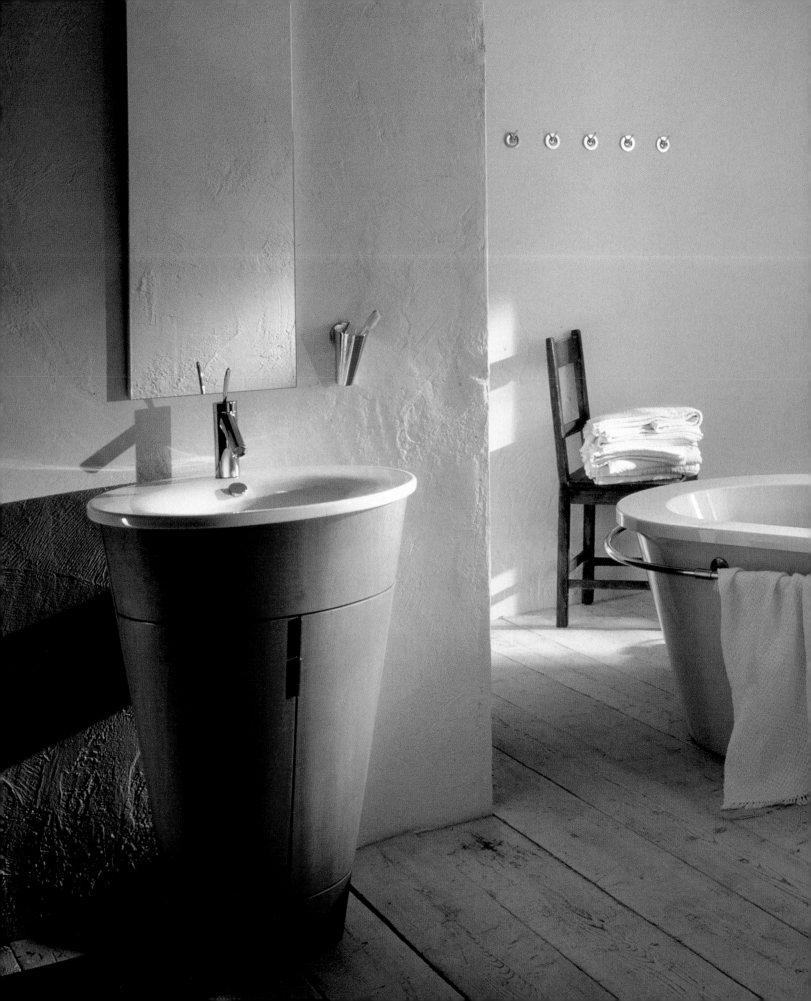

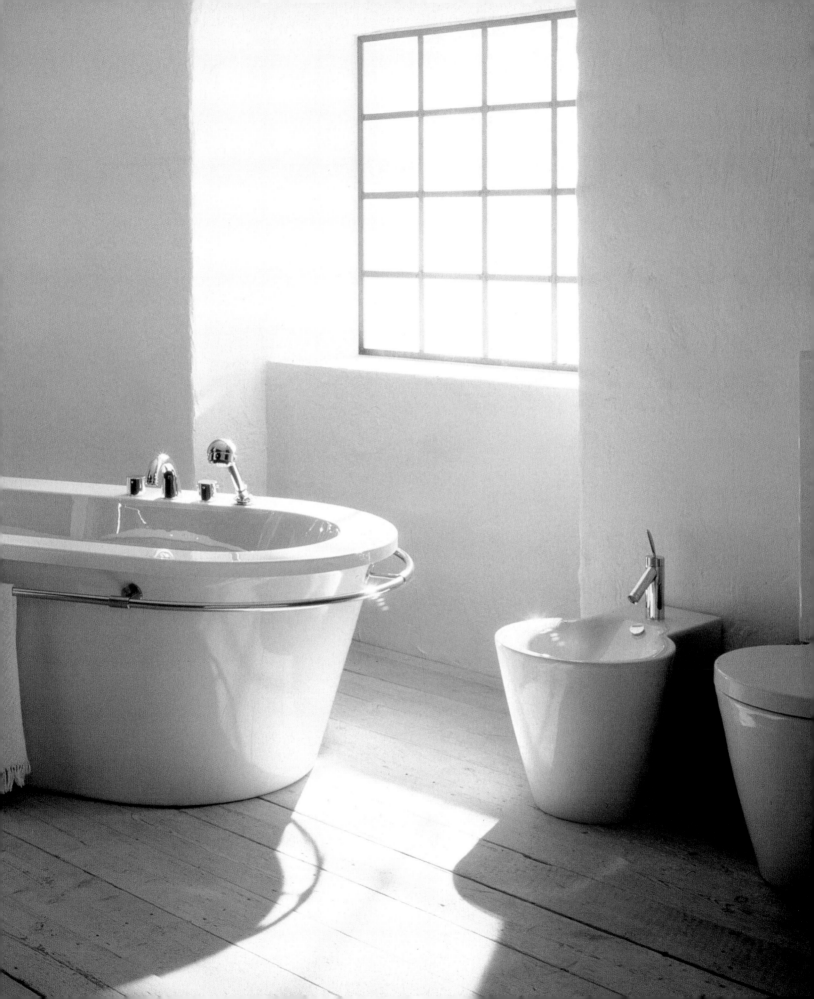

vering and wall tiles, should be a discreet backdrop that you can vary again and again very slightly with relatively small modifications – by means of curtains, mats, furniture, changing colours, accessories and plants. In this way you can experience one and the same bathroom again and again as if it were new.

Of course, this works best if the basic colour of the plumbing fixtures, floor and walls is kept a neutral shade. Pastel colours are the most favourable. With just a few decorations you can create very different moods. Of course, you must keep to a particular motif and then vary it imaginatively. A particular curtain and floor mat colour should perhaps be echoed in the other accessories, e.g. in the towels, flannels, flowers in the vase or the self-dyed bath salt in an attractive preparation jar. You do not need to throw this equipment away next time you change the scene. Simply stow them in the attic and get them out again next year.

Why not change the bathroom's appearance to fit in with the seasons? In spring it is the turn of pastel shades, yellow to orange, so as to echo the joy you feel with the passing of the winter. A colourful bunch of spring flowers on the windowsill, yellow foam plastic ducklings as bath sponges, bright yellow towels and orange flannels would serve the purpose well. Then follows the summer bathroom in bolder colours. The textiles convey a powerful red, in the vase are red roses, a cake of red soap is lying on the washbasin and the floor is covered with a new bath mat in a red pattern. For autumn, muted colours can be appropriate, russet brown or shades of purple, dried herbs in a bowl. And in the winter months, when the world outside loses its colours, you can introduce an iridescent blue into the bathroom, a hint of the sea, perhaps a fishing net on the ceiling, shells on the windowsill, a glass dolphin or two, little light blue and dark blue bottles containing bath essences, blue and white fabrics.

COLOURS HAVE AN EFFECT ON THE SOUL

Everyone knows that you can design with colours. But colours have much more far-reaching effects than people generally realise. With certain colours you can achieve certain effects. By consciously using colours, it is possible to influence not just psychological processes but also physical ones. And as the bathroom is supposed to be a paradise of well-being, it is very important to quite consciously use colours there. For this you must be familiar with the effects of the individual colours.

Remember: less is more. Do not cram every square inch full of implements – whether it be over the washbasin, on the windowsill or in other places. Leave a few tastefully chosen decorative objects to achieve the desired effect.

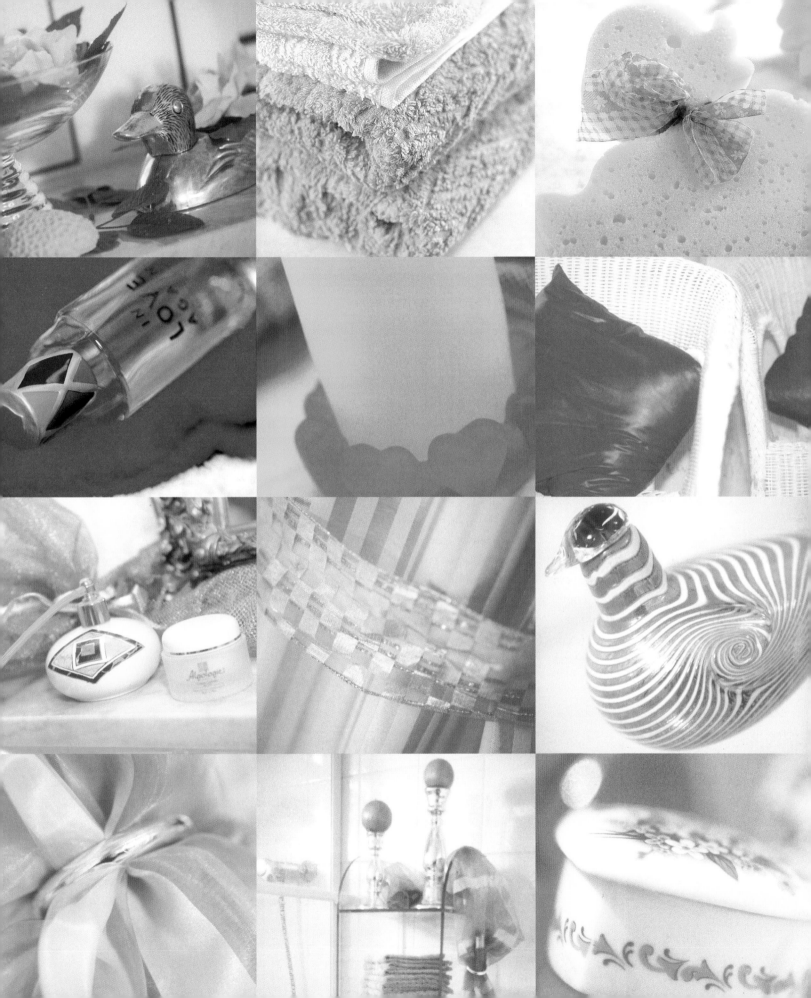

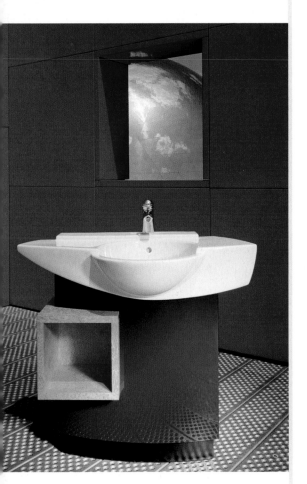

Red is the warmest colour, a colour full of energy; red is also the colour of fire. But you have to use the right dose of this colour. A red toothbrush tumbler in front of a white tiled wall has a stimulating effect, even though it is only a small spot of colour. Obviously this small amount of colour alone is sufficient to achieve such a conspicuously stimulating effect. By contrast, imagine a green toothbrush tumbler instead of the red one. You barely notice this colour combination. On the other hand, if you were to cover a whole wall with red tiles, the effect would be absolutely overpowering. The energy is simply too immense and it arouses the whole body. And that is certainly not intended in the bathroom – here you simply want to relax. You should just use red for particular emphasis. If you consider yourself to be more of a reserved type or perhaps find that you are even lacking in drive and are in need of more fire, intensify the emphasis on red.

There are of course colours that place limits on red and neutralise it. A door painted red surrounded by a relatively large wall covered with dark blue wallpaper loses a lot more of its vibrancy than if this red door were placed in white surroundings. When combined with the blue base of a washbasin, for example, a large red surface no longer has such an intense effect, although fiery red continues to dominate here of course.

Of course, shades of red can also be toned down and used to a more discreet effect. Light red is indeed still a stimulating colour, but it is not as overpowering as dark red. Pink tones certainly have a stimulating effect but in a much more enticing way. So if you place pink flowers in a vase in spring, you are transporting the budding force of the young season with all its freshness and exhilaration into the bathroom. In this way, you can feel spring directly.

Blue is a cool colour that brings vivacious natures down to earth and has a calming, soothing effect. Blue is the colour of the sea, evoking feelings of pensiveness, sorrow, melancholy and wanderlust. Such moods can easily give way to sadness – the "blues" – and this certainly would not boost your feeling of well-being in your private bathroom oasis.

Especially in smaller bathrooms, it is advisable to avoid using a lot of blue. A blue point of emphasis combined with red here and there may be favourable. Light blue, however, has a different effect. You could paint the ceiling in a light blue which would create a certain illusion of boundlessness – as if the bathroom were open to the sky. If, in addition, this blue background is shaped by spotlights, the little bathroom can suddenly burst its

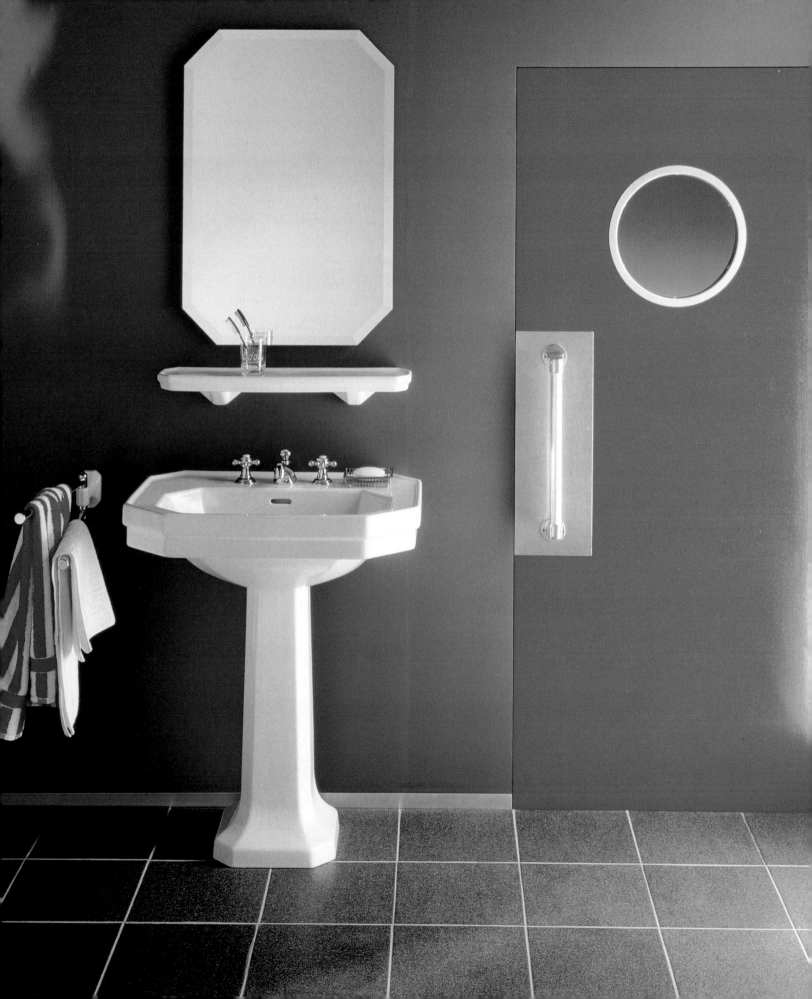

bounds. Keeping everything in a light blue tone – the floor and the walls – would definitely be too melancholic and could give off too much coldness. If you have everything blue, you would not be able to correct or supplement the colour scheme in a harmonious manner by emphasising other colours.

Yellow is a difficult, contrary colour if you consider its possible nuances. Yellow shades that are too intense, such as Indian yellow, chartreuse yellow, narcissus yellow or even lemon yellow, are irritating, make you nervous and dispel calmness. Aggressive colours are simply not suitable for a bathroom. On the other hand, all yellow tones that mix with red – such as orange, the soft colour of the complexion, the shimmer of gold that lies so beautifully on the body – are suitable because they put you in a good mood. Orange-coloured walls reflect this shade and thus also make the face and body enchanting if you look at yourself in the mirror or if you look at each other. A lovely, rich yellow lends the bathroom spaciousness, brings in the sun, warms the soul and mind and stimulates the metabolism. An appropriate yellow stimulates the hormonal balance and contributes greatly to the sense of well-being that everyone hopes to achieve when taking a bath.

Grey has a classic effect if it is not too dark, otherwise it can also easily result in dreariness if used to excess. Shades of grey may only be used very discreetly and always need an invigorating accent. Purple is particularly suitable for this, although you should not use it on large surfaces. A grey tiled floor, for example, creates a calming basis. If you then hang up some

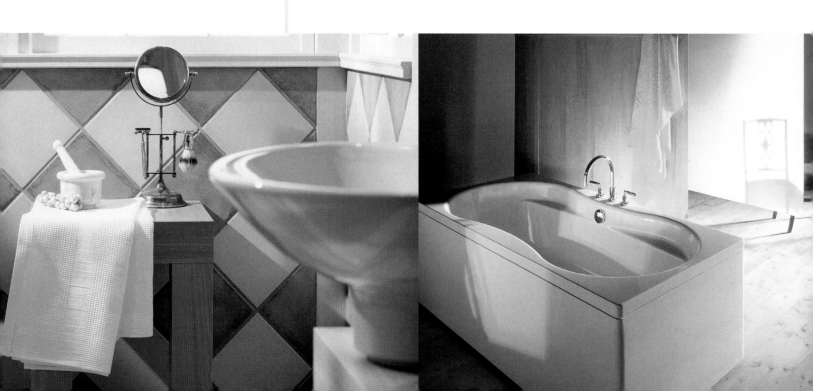

purple towels, you will create a wonderful harmony of colours that reaches to your very soul – all in all a princely, sublime feeling.

Green is generally regarded as a very pleasant, natural colour. It is considered to be the colour of hope, which comes from the fact that green is the dominant colour of living nature. Think about how the first little green shoots push up through the earth after a harsh winter, and when the fields and forests are then gradually transformed into green, this is synonymous with nature and life. Green makes you feel at peace and communicates cosiness. If you use green, it should be more in the direction of yellow and not be mixed too much with blue. A bilious green with too much blue content has a less pleasant effect. It should be the green of a delicious apple or a meadow, and in this instance you can also go through the whole range of green with the accessories. Shades of red do not harmonise with the calming nature of green. In this case, fire is the enemy of blossoming nature.

A white bathroom is still a classic. With white, you can lend an air of spaciousness even to small rooms that feel gloomy. White is boundless. But white also does larger rooms a lot of good. It is the colour of purity, it stands for light and life, gives you a liberating feeling and stimulates the breathing. A white bathroom does not have to be completely lacking in imagination; this depends on how you use other colour accents to brighten up the white surroundings. Basically you can use whatever colours appeal to you. Of course it is ideal to combine white tiles with pastel shades or even stronger colour patterns.

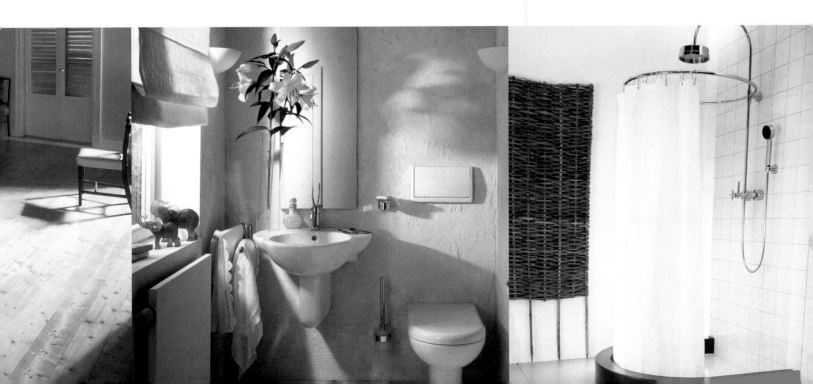

FENG SHUI FOR YOUR BATHROOM PARADISE

Feng Shui, if you translate it literally from Chinese, simply means "wind and water". Feng Shui is a doctrine that is thousands of years old and is concerned with the correct distribution of energy in a person's surroundings. The Chinese believe that a force exists that sets all life in motion and keeps it going. This force cannot be equated with physical quantities. It is a scientifically immeasurable vitality that however streams through all living things, including supposedly inanimate matter such as houses, rocks, mountains, valleys, rivers and the sea. The Chinese call this life force "chi". In this way, every individual human being is also filled with "chi" that constantly streams through the whole organism in harmonious movements. The energy of the environment is in a similar constant stream and harmonises with the internal flow of a human being.

It can happen that certain influences in the environment get in the way of this harmonious flow of energy. Energy blockages are the result, or to put it another way, human beings in such unfavourable energy situations do not feel at ease or indeed they even feel sick. So the art of Feng Shui involves formulating laws and deriving rules from them which – if correctly applied – ensure that such energy blockages are dispersed or do not arise in the first place.

The rules of Feng Shui can be applied to the whole design of our surroundings – the garden, the house and its individual rooms – and even on a much larger scale to the overall arrangement of the streets, houses and other buildings in a town. In this connection, however, we are only interested in how the rules of Feng Shui apply to the way the bathroom should be fitted out.

To our minds, which are more accustomed to logical thinking, Feng Shui appears at first glance to be mere superstition. And when, for example, in Hong Kong, you experience for yourself how rich people spend immense sums of money on having lucky numbers included on the registration plates of their cars, this impression seems to be confirmed. But if you take the trouble to analyse the ostensibly so irrational rules of Feng Shui to get down to the pragmatic crux, it quickly becomes clear that many pieces of Feng Shui advice find favour with our so-called common sense.

Feng Shui postulates, for example, that junk in a corner of a home destroys the flow of energy and therefore has a negative emotional effect on the residents. We would not put it this way, but would simply say that in such chaos you would feel uneasy and prefer to avoid such places. Why is this so? As an explanation we cite our aesthetic sense – such an untidy corner of waste troubles us or we even think of vermin settling in there, which could detract from life in the home.

It is exactly the same with another prime example of Feng Shui that we can also cite for the bathroom. The Chinese say that you always have to keep the toilet lid down because otherwise the energy will escape through it, which is tantamount to saying that all the residents' assets will end up in the lavatory. It is an open question whether this will really come true and harm the bank account of the residents. However, it is definitely a bad habit not to close the lid of the toilet. Evil smells spread and something can even fall into the toilet by accident, maybe a watch, and you then have to go to a lot of trouble to get it out of the water again. Apart from this, in a neat bathroom you often feel bothered if the open toilet is so obvious. So Feng Shui really does make sense and you can certainly consider the bathroom from these points of view.

The bath and the toilet have two very important functions for hygiene: they clean and relieve you, but these two places do not belong together. A shortage of living space or the desire of architects to make savings often result in the toilet being integrated into the bathroom. This in itself is a really impractical arrangement, as you like to use the bath for longish periods now and then and you generally do not mind if other members of the family go about their business there at the same time. But most people, of course, go to the toilet alone: when someone is lying in the bath for relaxation and enjoyment, the other person would feel very uneasy about using the toilet. So you can explain very pragmatically – and without the help of fictitious energy flows – Feng Shui's disquiet with regard to the placement of the toilet and bathtub together.

As a compromise solution for the bathroom with a toilet, Feng Shui suggests partitioning off the toilet where possible by means of a curtain or a screen – this could even be a relatively low pane of milk glass or a very narrow shelf as a room divider. Furthermore, Feng Shui forbids the practice of having the toilet bowl visible as soon as you open the bathroom door. Of course you can only avoid this if you are able to completely redesign your bathroom and if the circumstances in the room make it at all possible to conceal the toilet bowl in a corner.

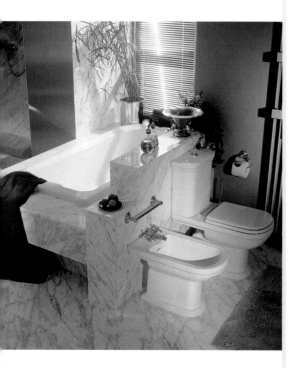

The bath and the toilet should be fairly clearly separated from the living area. This means that the sanitary area should be placed at the rear of the living space. To make such a separation really clear, you could draw a curtain in front of the bath-toilet area or install a folding door. It is disastrous for the bathroom and the toilet to be situated right at the entrance to the home. The first thing confronting anyone entering the house will be the ablutions area – bad smells and an unpleasant sight. On the other hand, anyone who has a home like this will just have to put up with it.

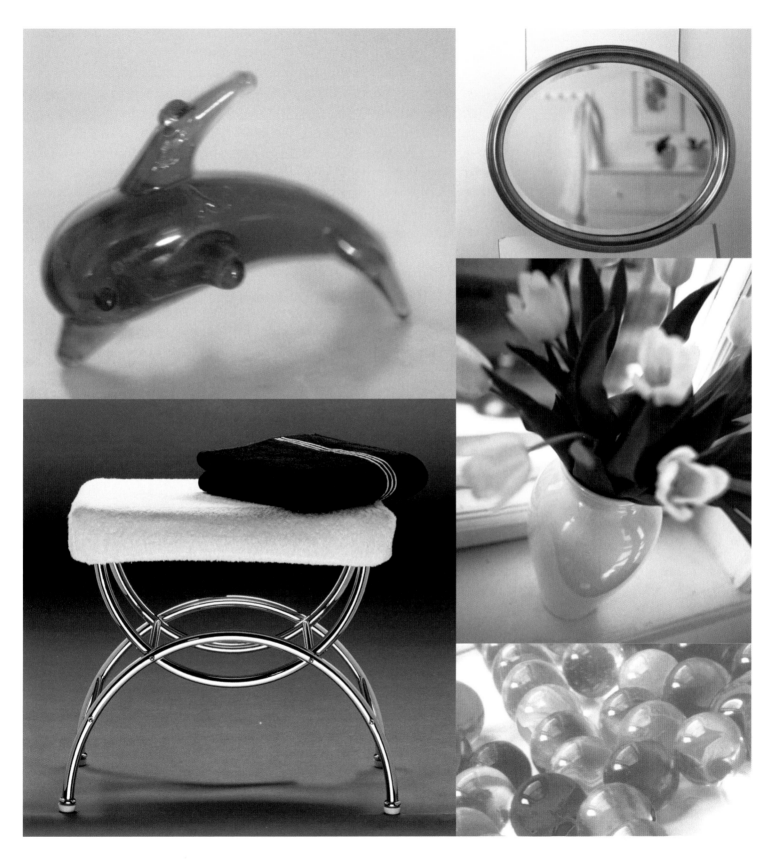

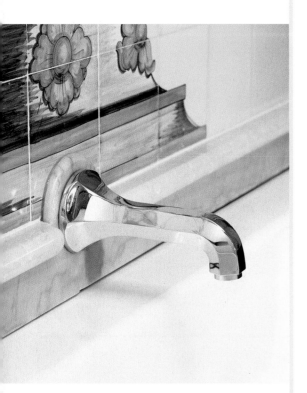

The only solution is for all members of the family to get used to leaving the door to this room closed. It is also helpful to ensure good automatic ventilation in the bathroom so that when you open the door (or forget to shut it occasionally) the smells from the toilet will not get into the rest of the living area. You can also combat the bad air with strong fragrant soap or a fragrance dish placed near the toilet bowl.

But you should also make sure the taps or the lavatory cistern do not drip or leak or that the drains are blocked. If this were the case, energy (in the dripping tap) would senselessly seep away or (in the case of a blocked drain) be prevented from flowing freely.

For a harmonious flow of energy, the bathroom needs a large window that lets a lot of energy, in the form of light, into the room. Dark colours devour energy – which is why Feng Shui urges you to concentrate on light colours. We have no trouble understanding this recommendation, either. Feng Shui also implies that the energy flows at excessive speed through a window without a curtain or accessories placed in front of it and so strikes people in the room too strongly. To reduce such peaks of energy, Feng Shui experts advise using thin colour-coordinated curtains or placing plants on the windowsill. We can also accept this stipulation because a large, bare window also makes us feel troubled, as it is uncovered and looks too bright. With even just one plant, the glass façade has a much more pleasant feel to it.

Feng Shui, however, only allows plants with round leaves, because elongated, pointed leaves or even the prickles of cactuses can shoot so-called poison arrows at people and thus disturb their energy balance. We can agree with this stipulation without reservation because you are mostly naked in the bathroom and pointed leaves and especially cactus spines can cause nasty injuries.

If your bathtub is directly in front of a very wide, high window and the bathroom door is positioned opposite, a Feng Shui expert will point out that there is too much energy and that it is also rushing in through the window too quickly and leaving the room again through the door without taking any detours, according to the law of the shortest path. Now anyone sitting in such a bath cannot feel completely at ease because the energy passing through is shaking up his or her inner energy balance. Feng Shui recommends reducing the flow of energy, diverting it and thus deflecting it into more pleasant circular movements which no longer disturb the per-

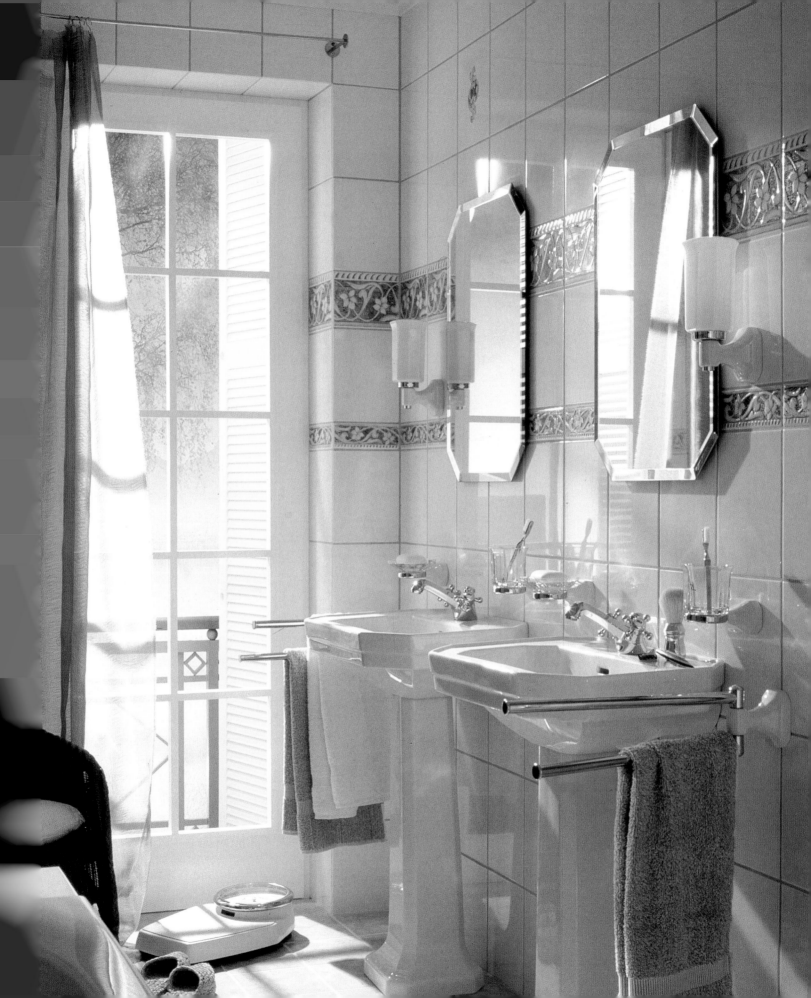

son sitting in the bath. This deflection can be in the form of a vase of flowers, decorative colourful bottles or a pot plant on the windowsill. It could also be a mobile or a set of tubular bells hanging over the window.

Fine curtains made of thin gossamer material can also subdue the flow of energy. It goes without saying that anyone sitting in the bath with closed eyes wanting to bask in it and enjoy the water will appreciate not being in a showcase in this situation. Even if no one is looking in through the large bare window, it will still somehow trouble you, whereas having accessories on the windowsill or over the window creates the feeling of being better screened from the outside.

Feng Shui believes in the use of additional specific aids such as rocks and crystals that are said to have energy and power. They are supposed to help neutralise negative energy flows and in this way keep harmful influences away from human beings. Crystals, according to Feng Shui, should always be cut symmetrically, since a lack of symmetry tips the energy out of balance. Precious stones should not be too large, otherwise they would concentrate too much energy, and this in turn has a disadvantageous effect.

Mirrors play a crucial role in directing energy. To our minds, if they are hung astutely, they can make even small rooms appear a great deal larger. Feng Shui argues that one or more mirrors send the energy to and fro and so they ensure vitality in rooms in which the energy would otherwise simply stagnate.

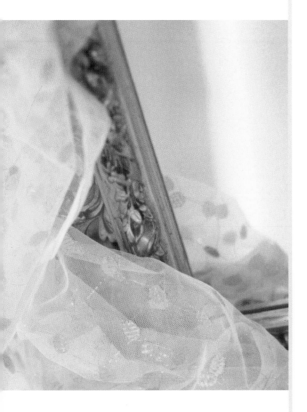

This is particularly the case in bathrooms without windows. Just imagine that you are entering a completely windowless bathroom and opposite the door are the washbasins with a mirror cabinet attached. The bathtub is positioned on the right. In this cramped room you can easily start to feel anxious. Now if the mirror situated opposite the door is very large and does not just show part of your face but also your body from head to waist, the room gains visually in breadth; in fact, it appears to be double the size. Whilst this is a mere illusion, you certainly feel this spaciousness as a relief.

Divided mirrors and mirror tiles that fragment your image are considered unfavourable. You could also say that they impair the illusion of the width of the room because their mosaic effect constantly signals that it is all just an optical illusion.

Taking a Bath Surrounded by Greenery

Many people dream of having a lovely big enamel bathtub in the garden, surrounded by a luxuriant jungle of plants. And there you would like to feel fantastic under the warming sun, whose light shimmers so mysteriously through the green of the leaves. Today people take it for granted that you have plants in your home and many people even arrange a real little garden on the windowsill. Now that the primitive shower corner has been turned into a cosily designed bathing temple in most households, plants are also gradually being smuggled into this living area.

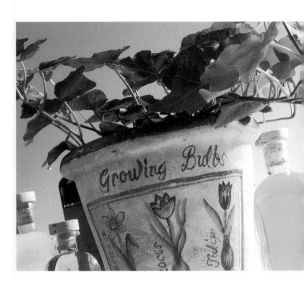

There is no question that plants are ideally suited to the bathroom. Where there is water there is life, and plants quite naturally belong there too. Of course, you cannot put just any plant in the bathroom because extreme conditions prevail there at times. But a row of green blossoming plants certainly gives you a very good feeling in the bathroom, too. You just have to select them carefully according to the conditions that prevail in this environment.

Light is sometimes a problem. Plants cannot thrive in a windowless room; light is essential for them. They need light the whole year through and for a relatively long period of time. Temperature is an additional problem, which is why not all plants are suitable for the bathroom. Here mostly relatively high temperatures prevail. Temperatures of 25 °C (77 °F) and above are not uncommon. Plants that are accustomed to lower temperatures are therefore out of the question. In the bathroom temperatures often fluctuate widely. When the bathing session is over, the window is opened wide to let out the steam and most people also turn off the heating because they do not want to heat the room unnecessarily twenty-four hours a day. For the plants, this means quite a drop in temperature, especially in winter, when after a hot steamy bath hour, icy cold air suddenly streams in the window. This is a shock to sensitive plants.

In other words, you have to select plants that are not bothered much by these extreme temperatures because they are by nature so robust. On the other hand, when you are airing the room you should also be considerate and in the winter you could perhaps have regular minimum heating and not be too extreme in ventilating the room. When you air it, you should not leave the plants near the window. So if you normally place them on the windowsill, you will have to move them elsewhere while you are airing the room.

Understandably, the humidity of the air in the bathroom is very high. But all plants that originally come from humid climatic zones will experience this as pleasant.

The choice of plants also depends on their individual growth rhythms. As the temperature conditions described prevail in the bathroom all year round, plants with specific dormant periods are out of the question – they cannot be placed in the bathroom on a permanent basis. In spite of all these limiting factors, there is a wide range of suitable plants, particularly foliate plants.

You will not have to worry much about pests and diseases, and in living areas fungal diseases are seldom encountered. However, as already mentioned, damage can arise due to the shock effect of extreme differences in temperature.

The following green plants come into consieration: ornamental asparagus (Asparagus densiflorus), an especially robust plant for bathrooms that are not too hot, various species of the leafy begonia (Chlorophytum comosum), especially the spider plant that is suitable as a hanging plant, the kangaroo vine (Cissus antarctica), and the grape ivy (Cissus rhombifolia), which is suitable as a hanging plant or creeper. For getting through a winter that is none too warm, various species of the lemon are suitable, in particular the especially robust reed grass (Cyperus alternifolius), which requires a great deal of moisture. The dieffenbachia needs a lot of light. There is also ivy, a climbing and hanging plant that makes few demands, and various species of the dwarf pepper (Peperomia) that likes being kept rather moist although it cannot tolerate too much dampness. The philodendron, the pilea and maidenhair grass (Scirpucernuus) and the baby's tears also fit well into your bathroom scenery. The following seed plants are recommended: Athurium scherzerianum hybrids such as the flamingo plant, the African violet, the leafy vexillum (do not let it get too hot!) and various bromeliads (bromelias).

You will not have any problems with cut flowers, which you can of course arrange in a vase in the bathroom. Cut flowers naturally introduce very imaginative colours to the décor, and especially if you want to vary the bathroom from time to time you can achieve a highly decorative effect with seasonal garlands of flowers. You can position small vases in various places where there is only room for a few or even just individual flowers. But you can also place a large floor vase in a corner, with a really beautiful bunch of flowers.

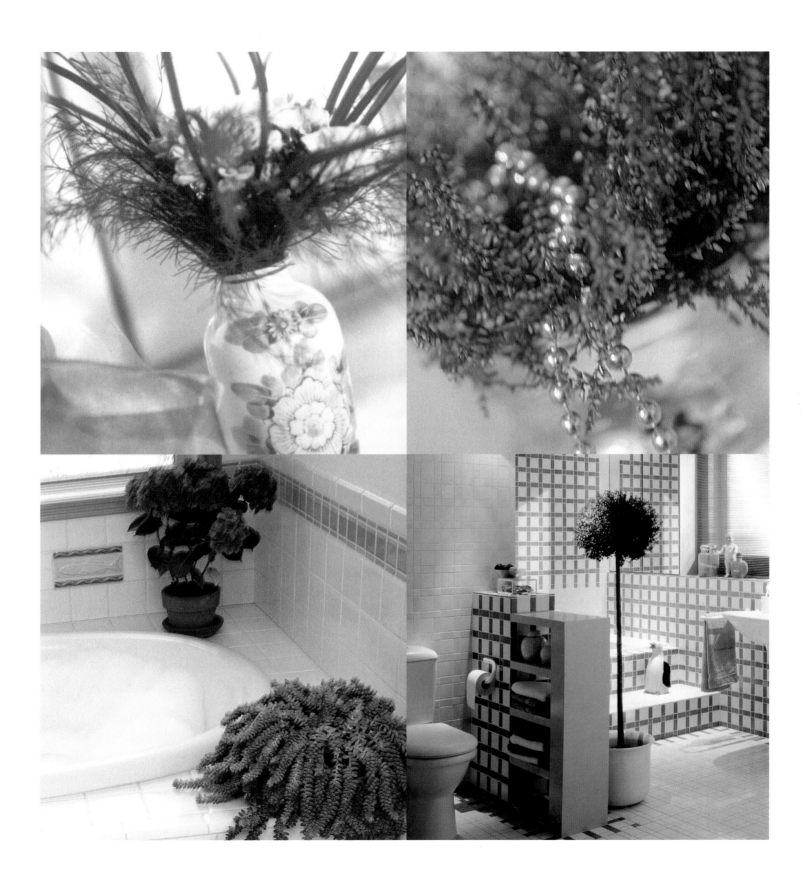

INDEX

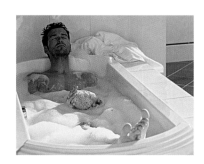